Another Day

Also by Pat Seed

ONE DAY AT A TIME

Another Day

PAT SEED MBE

Foreword by
HRH The Duchess of Kent

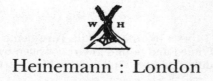

Heinemann : London

98302219

William Heinemann Ltd
10 Upper Grosvenor Street,
London W1X 9PA

LONDON   MELBOURNE   TORONTO
JOHANNESBURG   AUCKLAND

First published in Great Britain 1983
Copyright © Pat Seed 1983

434 67862 7
L000261459

Typeset by Inforum Ltd, Portsmouth
Printed and bound in Great Britain by
Biddles Limited, Guildford & King's Lynn

For my dear husband, Geoffrey,
without whose encouragement,
none of this would have been possible.

Foreword by
HRH The Duchess of Kent

SHE IS A wife – as many are. She is a mother – as many are. She is a woman who works – as many are. She is inextricably involved in family and friends – as many are. She has been faced with the fear of pain, illness and death – as many are. This is the ordinary side of Pat Seed.

The extraordinary side is that she has become a mirror for her own philosophy of 'One day at a time' and that in this mirror literally millions have seen an image of themselves which gives new strength, hope and courage.

Following the first account which Pat Seed gave of her cancer challenge, she now gives the story of her own successful medical treatment for cancer.

It is the story of an indomitable crusade against an illness which is universally feared carried on by one woman with many willing helpers.

As her days – one day at a time – continue to unfold they provide a continuing illustration and inspiration to humanity that all have within reach the means to overcome difficulty and disease.

From personal experience Pat Seed can now share the good news that cancer can be medically treated. But she does much more than that – she provides a key to what unites humanity because her life illustrates fundamental principles which have no frontiers.

Katharine

September 21st 1982.

1

MY HUSBAND GEOFFREY stood on the spectators' balcony at Manchester Airport, watching the plane gaining height and eventually become a microscopic dot in the sky before it was obscured by cloud. It was at this moment that he wondered what on earth he'd been thinking of, to allow his wife to make a ten day transatlantic trip when she was a woman suffering from cancer.

But it was too late now for second thoughts. Pauline and I were on our way. Even Concorde couldn't beat it – just a fraction of a second on my ciné film – to cross the Atlantic. One sequence is the aerial view over Prestwick and the next shot is of the water-logged approach to J.F. Kennedy airport. In fact, typical of the amateur movie maker.

For Pauline and I it was our first trip to the United States and we could hardly believe it was happening. If it wasn't for that ciné record and a few souvenirs, there are times when we wonder if it did happen.

The purpose of our visit was to see at close quarters the prototype of an inanimate object which had occupied my every waking thought since January 1977 – the Emiscanner 7070, a highly sophisticated piece of British technology which held out new hope for cancer patients. It was in January 1977 that I was given the medical prognosis of six months to live. Coming to terms with the fact that you have cancer and not much of a future takes some doing, but you have no choice. I had picked myself up off the floor, had tried to discipline myself to living 'one day at a time' and I had also got my dander up – good and proper – and had fought back in as practical a way as I knew.

At the Christie Hospital and Holt Radium Institute, Manchester, Europe's largest cancer treatment centre, there was much shaking of heads. Here was a painfully thin female patient telling them she was going to raise the money for a piece of equipment which the N.H.S. couldn't afford to provide. As the sum needed at that time was half a million pounds, it is small wonder that the hospital staff thought they'd got a nut case as well as a terminal cancer patient on their hands. If they – or I – had then known that the initial figure would treble, I doubt whether what came to be known as 'The Scanner Trail' would ever have taken its first few faltering steps.

Refusing to be 'written off', I did some stocktaking. The debit side was bleak, but what was there on the credit side? I am happily married and surrounded by a loving and very supportive family. I am a journalist, therefore I have knowledge of the communications media. I have previous experience of charity work and know how a charity should be organised and what pitfalls are to be avoided. I have a strong faith in the teaching of Jesus Christ. To add to the cards in my hand is my sense of humour which is often my undoing and sometimes the joker running wild. All of these would have been enough to found a charity but fate had given me an added impetus – first hand experience of cancer.

And so on 15th March 1977, two days before my 49th birthday the Pat Seed Appeal Fund was launched. I sought the help of other journalists on newspapers and those working for radio and television knowing full well that the story of a dying woman who was trying to raise money for a machine which could help other patients, but not herself, was a good one.

There followed two incredibly eventful years. My Appeal caught the imagination of a generous-hearted British public; I found myself working a sixteen hour day, dealing with the administrative side of the Fund; clocking up endless miles on motorways; attending functions, rallying support especially in the North West of England. In the process I made a whole host of new friends and became so busy that I had little time to dwell on the state of my own health.

I had a Central Committee of the Fund, under the chairmanship of Sir William Downward, Lord Lieutenant of Greater Manchester, whose members included three of the consultants of the Christie. And there were to be sixty-eight local fund-raising committees throughout the vast region served by the Christie. A truly great team. It's one thing to have a good idea, but you need an awful lot of help to enable you to reach a goal of such magnitude. That help had been forthcoming from every quarter and from all sections of society; from members of the Royal Family, from people in every walk of life, from children and from old age pensioners. To me, it was nothing less than a miracle. For exactly two years to the day since I had walked out of the Christie having been told I'd 'had it' I had laid the foundation stone for the new Department of Computerised Axial Tomography at the hospital. There to help me do it were an old age pensioner and a child, representing the entire age range of the people who had made it possible.

To my great delight, the inventor of the Scanner, Nobel Prize winner Dr Godfrey Hounsfield, was there to make sure that stone was well and truly laid. It was a time for celebration and a time for thanksgiving. Six months to live? Two years had passed and I was still doing my damndest to stay alive. There was still so much to be done.

A few days later, the manuscript of my first book *One Day At a Time* was in the hands of the publishers. The story of my 'scanner trail', it tells the story of the appeal – the humour, headaches and heartaches and of the people, famous and

3

not so well known, who filled it full of laughter and tears and helped to provide the happy ending.

What more could I want?

To see that scanner!

In case I wouldn't be around long enough to see the building completed (in January 1979 the site looked like Steptoe's yard) and the scanner installed at the Christie, EMI Medical had generously offered to fly me out to their Chicago factory where 'our' scanner was to be assembled and also to the Mallinckrodt Institute of Radiology in St Louis, Missouri where the prototype was being put through its paces.

That was why, on 7th March 1979 my very dear friend Pauline Heaton, the Appeal Fund Secretary and I found ourselves airborne aboard a Super VC 10 en route from Manchester Airport bound for New York. The Manchester based crew and hostesses looked after us admirably, had a 'whip round' for my Fund, and the Captain honoured us by inviting us on to the flight deck.

When friends knew of our USA trip, some had grinned and said: 'Uncle Sam doesn't know what he's letting himself in for!' It took me exactly ten minutes on American soil to prove them right.

In the foyer of J.F. Kennedy airport, I stood with our cases and paraphernalia at my feet as Pauline went outside in search of a yellow cab. A porter asked me if I wanted the baggage trucking outside, to which I replied a grateful 'Yes please'. When it was stowed away in the cab, it suddenly occurred to me that he would expect a tip. I searched frantically in my handbag, found my purse and looked with dismay at the unfamiliar United States coins. I had no idea, at that point, what any of them were worth. Hastily selecting the largest silver coin in the collection, I gave it to him, smiled 'thank you' and got in the cab. As Pauline was about to sit beside me, the man looked at the coin in disgust and said, 'here, lady, have it back!'

Oh heavens! Gaffe number one. I emptied the coins on

4

my lap and when we had worked out their values, I realised
that I had given him the American equivalent of $2\frac{1}{2}$p. No
wonder he had looked disgusted for he would expect at least
a dollar. Eventually, the cab drew up in front of our hotel on
West 44th Street, Manhattan. We probably over compensated when we tipped the driver, for he looked as pleased as
if he'd just won a State Lottery.

As we entered the hotel, I grinned at Pauline. 'We'll have
to shape better than that. D'you remember Mark Twain's
"Innocents Abroad"? I dare say that by the end of this trip,
we would be able to give him enough material for another
book, were he still alive!'

For business reasons, we were four days in New York
before flying on to Chicago. Before our USA visit I had
contacted a journalist friend who was doing a one year
course at Columbia University. He had written to say that
New York weather was arctic and to be sure to bring warm
clothing. This had prompted my worried Mother to insist
that I borrow her fur coat. I could have wished that fur coat
far enough, for when Robin met us the following day he told
us that the glorious warm sunshine was the city's first taste of
Spring.

Manhattan seemed hard, noisy, bustling and impersonal.
One felt that if one dropped down dead, nobody would bat
an eyelid. They'd just step over the body and leave it for
some other guy to see that the pieces ended up in the right
trash can. Yet it was fascinating to see at close quarters,
scenes and places one had only seen before by courtesy of
Hollywood or television. We were left with a kaleidoscope of
fleeting impressions; the view from the top of the World
Trade Centre giving panoramic vistas in every direction
and with the Statue of Liberty, looking positively microscopic, perched on the outcrop of rock where the waters of
the Hudson and East River meet.

We also took the elevator to the top of the Rockefeller
Centre. As it begins the ascent, a recorded commentary
starts. It ends as the doors open just 58 seconds later on the

5

70th floor with the words 'mind your step'. At that height, what choice is there? On the roof of the building, we sat for a while in the spring sunshine. Looking over the balustrade at the scenes below with the congestion of traffic looking like a set of Dinkie cars, the term 'concrete jungle' seemed an apt description, for huge skyscrapers were cheek by jowl and every inch of available space seemed to have some building on it. If Manhattan wasn't built on granite bedrock, the whole lot would have sunk into the Hudson years ago. But the view of the Manhattan skyline from the Staten Island ferry is a view not to be missed. It is breathtaking. New York is really a series of islands linked together by vast bridges. We came to the conclusion that whoever decided on this location for a city must have liked doing things the hard way. New York is also hard on your feet. A bad attack of shingles along the entire length of my right leg has left me with an impaired sciatic nerve. Result – my brain doesn't always tell my leg what it is supposed to do. To sit down for a while became a necessity.

At a small movie theatre near the Rockefeller Centre, they were showing James Herriot's *All Creatures Great and Small*. I'd wanted to see the film back home, but I'd never found an opportunity. So for a couple of hours, there we were, in the middle of Manhattan, revelling in the beauty and serenity of the Yorkshire Dales.

Only two days away from U.K. and we were filled with nostalgia. Sitting in front of us were two American ladies. The film progressed to the part where James attends a sick goat and the farmer informs him dismally: 'It's eaten me summer drawers.' One of the American ladies drawled: 'What are drawers? Are they dusters?' I resisted the temptation to reply in broadest Lancashire 'No, luv, but they'll be fit for nowt else when t'goat's finished wi' 'em!'

Next morning, we were heading for Newark Airport, New Jersey for our flight to Chicago. It was Sunday and the four days in New York had passed all too swiftly. There was so much we hadn't had time to see. We had had a small bite at 'The Big Apple' but not a big enough bite to know whether we would eventually grow to love the flavour.

Now we were heading by DC10 to O'Hare Airport, reputedly the biggest and busiest airport in the world. As the plane circled to land, Lake Michigan stretched into infinity and it was frozen as far as the eye could see. Apart from that vast expanse of ice, it reminded me of the front at Blackpool, except that Blackpool's Tower would have looked puny in comparison to the one at which we were now looking – the Sears Tower, over a quarter of a mile high and the world's tallest building.

As we came through the airport terminal there to greet us was the friendly familiar face of Trevor Perry, EMI's U.K. North West representative.

The Alcarres Restaurant, north of Chicago . . . delectable food, excellent service and a luxurious decor. Huge picture windows afforded panoramic views of the pastoral scene beyond. A bridge over a gently meandering stream and its snow covered banks, overhung with frost laden trees sparkling in the sunshine. It was a winter wonderland and could have been the setting for a Hollywood movie. It used to be Al Capone's hideaway. When things got too hot for him in the city, he holed up here until the heat was off. Had it been like this in his day, he'd surely never have left it to go stirring up chaos in Chicago and the city might not have acquired the reputation for being a town of hoodlums and gangsters. If there were any around on that pleasant Sunday afternoon, they must have been having a siesta, for we didn't meet any. Yet evidence that they still exist was on the exterior of the Police Headquarters, which was hung with black and purple drapings in silent tribute to three murdered policemen.

Fortunately, Pauline Heaton and I saw Chicago from the safety and comfort of a chauffeur driven Cadillac and in the company of a member of EMI staff. The city is smaller, yet more spacious than New York and has a beautifully landscaped frontage onto the shore of Lake Michigan. It boasts the world's largest post office, the world's largest hotel (The Conrad Hilton) and has the headquarters of a famous brand of chewing gum. Tom, our driver was a Chicagoan of Irish extraction and he told us that on St Patrick's Day, they dye the Chicago River green. A delightful character and full of Irish charm, this former fireman showed us the sights – the famous Loop railway (reminiscent of Liverpool's dockland overhead railway); the Magnificent Mile, Chinatown with its pagoda roofed telephone kiosks and he pointed out some of Chicago's famous stores and nightspots.

The following morning, we visited the Northbrook factory of EMI Medical Incorporated which is the sister company of EMI UK Medical. Here, we saw scanners in various stages of assembly and some crated ready for shipment to hospitals in all parts of the world. We began to appreciate why this sophisticated technology cost so much money.

After lunch, we were airborne again heading in a DC9 for St Louis and the Mallinckrodt Institute of Radiology. Here, we saw the prototype of EMI's electronic masterpiece, the Emiscanner 7070. This was the main purpose of our trip for the next machine off the production line was earmarked for the Christie Hospital, Manchester, and would be the first of its kind in Europe. It would be the tangible result of the hard work of a multitude of caring people who had provided the money. I am not ashamed to admit that, as I watched an elderly patient being scanned I felt very emotional. Behind that fibre glass casing is a complicated mass of computerised wizardry. A three second scan through a cross section of the body (a 'slice') picks up one and a half *million* readings which the computers convert and present as a picture on a TV screen on the console – in just *forty seconds* and with a clarity of detail far in advance of those produced by earlier models. Press the appropriate buttons and the computer prints out a stream of information on the other of the twin screens, as plus or minus numerals.

8

Having LIVED 'scanner' for the past two years, this was for me the highlight of the trip. At last, I had actually *seen* the thing for which I'd been working.

In a waiting room, I talked to an elderly man marked out for radiotherapy. Around his throat were purple gentian lines, marking the tumour site. Knowing that America has nothing like our British National Health Service, I asked him what it was going to cost him.

'Oh, about 2,000 dollars, I guess.'

'Have you got that kind of money, or are you insured?'

'No, I'm not insured, but I guess I'd have paid in about 2,000 dollars by now, if I had been. You take the chance on it.'

It certainly made me appreciate our Health Service. I shuddered to think what my own treatment must have cost. O.K., so it may not be a perfect service, but nobody in the United Kingdom goes short of treatment because they cannot afford to pay for it.

We left the hospital in time to take a quick look at St Louis before the daylight waned.

Until the Louisiana Purchase Treaty of 1803, St Louis was little more than a stockaded fur trading outpost. It suddenly found itself the gateway to the west as more than a million square miles was added to the newly independent United States and settlers moved west along trails blazed by the old pioneers. This little outpost where the waters of the Missouri river and the mighty Mississippi join, became a thriving city. To commemorate St Louis' place in history, it now has one of the most breathtaking memorials to be erected by man. The Gateway Arch is a stainless steel structure which can be seen from a distance of thirty miles. Incredibly elegant and graceful its surfaces mirror the constantly changing cloudscapes, the sunshine or the moonlight and the night lights of the city. It weighs 16,678 tons and the distance across the base is the same as the height – 630 feet. You could put Blackpool Tower underneath it and still have about a hundred feet to spare. It is also known as

'The New Spirit of St Louis'. Moored alongside the levee at its base are some of the old showboats, most of which are now floating restaurants. Further down river is what was Mark Twain's home and the setting for *Tom Sawyer* and *Huckleberry Finn*.

As we left St Louis early on Tuesday morning, we saw, suspended from the ceiling of the airport foyer, the original Spirit of St Louis, the tiny monoplane in which Lindbergh flew the Atlantic. It is such a small, frail craft in which this courageous aviator made his historic journey.

Back at O'Hare airport we boarded a Boeing 707 for the next stage of our journey, this time to Montreal. Pauline went to see her brother and his family and I spent a few days with my cousin Peter and his family. Peter is a doctor at McGill University, engaged in cancer research. We had plenty to talk about, both family affairs and of the progress being made in the treatment of various forms of cancer. He and his wife Sue made me so welcome and the warmth of their hospitality more than made up for the 20 below zero temperatures in and around Montreal. Spring hadn't reached there yet.

All too soon, Pauline and I met at Montreal air terminal and as the huge 747 Jumbo took off just before midnight on 16th March, we reflected on the various aspects of our ten day whirlwind trip – six flights and goodness knows how many thousands of miles.

Somewhere over the Atlantic, watching the dawn rise, I said:

'D'you suppose it's my birthday?'

I was born on 17th March and being none too sure about the time factor, I really didn't know just when the date changed.

'Never mind. Let's celebrate anyway,' said Pauline and we ordered a couple of drinks on the strength of it.

When the plane landed at Heathrow on the morning of 17th March, there was the best sight I'd seen in ten days. My husband Geoff, with a welcoming grin on his face and waiting to give me a hug and a kiss.

England, blessed England . . . there's no place like home.

Along with Pauline and her husband and two daughters, we spent the weekend at Roy's London flat for I had an interview with Anna Ford scheduled for Monday morning. Roy Fisher is a Trustee of the Appeal Fund and one of our oldest and dearest friends. Geoff and I are godparents to his elder daughter, Susan.

To be screened by Thames TV during Easter Week, it was one of a series of interviews with people who had faced some kind of crisis in their life — and learned how to cope.

The following day, Geoff and I travelled north to Garstang and we had not been in the house more than a few minutes when the 'phone rang. It was a reporter from Manchester's Piccadilly Radio.

Had I heard the news?

'What news?'

'Oh . . . then I had better not say anything until you hear about it from the proper quarter. But you are in for a nice surprise. I'll come back to you later.'

With that I was left wondering. A few minutes later, a call came from Alan Ward, President of the Manchester Junior Chamber of Commerce to tell me that I had been chosen as 'Mancunian of the Year, 1979'.

Manchester City Council had already seen fit to give a civic reception in my honour. Now, the city of my birth and teenage years was about to honour me again. I felt very proud indeed.

But after the events of the last two weeks, my brain felt addled and I was tired out.

The Mancunian of the Year staggered upstairs, flopped into bed and went out like a light.

2

PAULINE AND FAMILY had returned from London on Sunday. For her daughters and for Neville, her headmaster husband, Monday meant 'back to school'. On Wednesday, the pair of us set about tackling the amount of mail which had accumulated during our absence. Within no time at all the USA trip might never have been. We were back in the old routine.

At the Christie, to my untrained eye, the building site looked an utter shambles, yet to the architects and builders it was all part of the master plan and they assured me the building would be ready by the autumn when our scanner was due to arrive.

I was terribly keyed up, impatient for it all to be fact, at long last, instead of an impossible dream. I was nervous, too, about *One Day At a Time*, due to be published in the autumn. Some people take years to write a book. This one had been written in six weeks. I'd come off the 'scanner trail' in the middle of December and got down to writing. With the family Christmas thrown in for good measure, I'd finished it by the end of January 1979, which was the publishers' deadline. Most journalists are used to writing under pressure, and I'd never failed to meet a deadline yet. Now I was full of doubts, second thoughts, alternating between a kind of nervous excitement at the thought of becoming an author and wondering if I could have made a better job of it

12

but for that remorseless enemy, time. However, for better or worse, the thing was done. Best forget it until the autumn. Worrying wouldn't help.

Worry comes in all shapes and sizes. In February 1979, Bob Atkinson, the son of the President of Barrow-in-Furness Soroptimists had decided to do a marathon run from Barrow Town Hall to my home in Garstang in celebration of his 21st birthday. On the 15th, Pauline and I drove to Manchester in a Ford Capri, lent to me by my local garage, whilst my Fiesta was being serviced. Driving back home in the late afternoon on the M61 was a nightmare.

All the gadgets were in a different place from those on my own car and we were almost back in Garstang before I discovered where the windscreen washer pump was located. On the motorway, a blizzard was obscuring all three lanes. One could only follow the driver in front and hope to heaven he could see better than I could. He, in turn, was probably relying on the driver in front of *him*. It was a slow cautious crawl, when quick brake application could have meant disaster. Thankfully, we arrived home safely. Although concentrating on driving, I had been worrying about Bob and his marathon. That evening I telephoned him, suggesting that he postpone it until weather conditions were more suitable, but apparently the weather in Barrow wasn't all that bad.

'For goodness sake don't take any risks, Bob.'

I must have sounded like a mother hen. He laughed.

'Pat, stop worrying, I'll be just fine. In any case, my support group will be with me.'

Sixty miles seems an awfully long way, especially to someone like me who couldn't run ten yards without falling flat on her face.

'What time do you expect to arrive?'

'At about 4 p.m. I should think'.

The following morning a thought struck me. I knew that Bob would want a hot bath and a change of clothing and I intended to give him a meal.

13

'Support group? How many people d'you suppose that will be?'

'Your guess is as good as mine,' said Pauline.

'Well, that's a fat lot of help! What's a meal that will stretch among a few extra folk, if need be? – I know, Lancashire hot pot. Warm, tasty and nourishing.' I abandoned the original menu and as there wasn't time to thaw out meat from the freezer, I dashed down to the butchers, bought a couple of pounds of beef, came home, put it to cook in the pressure cooker and then made two enormous apple pies. We knocked off for a bite of lunch and then my dear secretary abandoned her typewriter. We set about the vegetables – ten pounds of potatoes and plenty of carrots and onions.

I have an enormous hot pot dish made of brown earthenware; it is the type one uses for church or W.I. hot-pot suppers. This, with an outsize casserole dish would cope with the lot. At 2.30, just when the kitchen was looking like a disaster area and we were nearly ankle deep in potato peelings, there was a ring at the front door.

It can't be!

But it was.

'Don't let anyone in that kitchen!'

I opened the door and standing on the doorstep was a lithe young man wearing running shorts and vest and a broad grin of triumph. He'd run the sixty miles in record time.

'I've done it.'

'Well done. Well done, indeed, Bob. Come in.'

He came in, followed by three strapping men in track suits, four young ladies (presumably their girl friends) Vera, his mother, (Vera Atkinson, a super lass) and one of her friends, plus the photographer from the *Barrow News and Mail*.

I ushered them into the lounge and they sat down.

'You are earlier than I expected. There's hot pot and apple pie lined up for you at about five o'clock,' I told them.

'Meanwhile, we'll have a cup of tea.'

'Oh, don't worry about food,' said Vera. 'We wouldn't expect you to feed us all. A cup of tea will be fine. Then if Bob could have a quick bath, we'll be on our way.'

It seemed their back-up van had enough food to see them about as far as Katmandu! The photographer wanted to take pictures of Bob running down the drive, but as the Gas Board men had turned up the previous day, dug a channel down the length of the front lawn and left yellow flashing lights at intervals, I vetoed that one. However, there were plenty of alternatives.

We chatted over cups of tea and how the time flew by. We arranged that in the near future, when Bob had collected all his sponsor money, I would visit them in Barrow-in-Furness. Just after four, they left to drive back home. Bob had made a truly splendid contribution, but I was left with a problem. 'What on earth do I do with all this hot pot?'

There was enough to feed a regiment. Eventually, it was packed in the freezer in portions for two. On our return from America, Geoff and Mike told us that they had struggled manfully to get through as much of it as possible, but right now, the very thought of hot pot was enough to put them on hunger strike.

In May at Barrow Town Hall, Bob presented me with a cheque for £1,700 for the Fund. It was typical of the generosity of the people of Barrow-in-Furness. Later, we all went to Vera's house for a buffet supper which was delicious, but I couldn't resist telling the Mayor how near he'd come to having hot pot for his supper!

Talking of generosity, in February I was presented with a most beautiful gift. An original design and an exquisite piece of craftmanship, it is a sterling silver rose bowl in the shape of an open rose. Inscribed 'The Manchester Rose' it is a present from a group of Manchester people who were helping the Fund and is a token of their affection for me. Much as I treasure my lovely rose bowl, I value the affection with which it was given far more. Sometime in the future, I hope it will find a permanent home in Manchester Cathedral as tangible evidence of the goodwill which Mancunians have demonstrated, not just to me personally, but in their generous support of the Fund.

April 6th and the proofs of my book arrived. It had made up into 284 pages and the publishers wanted the corrected proofs returned as soon as possible. Then a phone call informed me that they would like them by return of post. Oh, heavens! How on earth do you proof read a book in 24 hours?

'Geoff, you'd better read this. If there's anything you think ought to come out, now is the time to say so. Once these proofs go back it will be too late.'

None of my family had read the book in manuscript form. If I was putting my heart on paper, it had to be *my* thoughts, *my* words. Geoff sat up into the small hours of the morning to finish it. As he was reading, I was like a cat on hot bricks.

When he had read the final page, I tentatively asked, 'Well?' He put his arms round me and kissed me.

'Don't change a word of it. That book is going to be of help to many people.'

I burst into tears. Geoff had lived through it all with me. He'd backed me up, encouraging me every step of the way. None of it would have happened without his love for me, his patient understanding, his reasoning integral sense of right and wrong and a logical approach which so often curbs my impetuosity. Can you wonder that I fought tooth and nail to stay alive? If Geoff approved of *One Day At a Time* that was good enough for me.

Although I corrected as many of the printing errors as possible, there were one or two which escaped notice, but there just wasn't time for a second scrutiny. In any case, on 7th April, Pauline and I were due in Oxford, where I was to be one of the speakers at the Royal College of Nursing Oncology Conference. Oncology being the study of malignant diseases, all the nurses attending were involved in the care of cancer patients. As well as professional speakers, a

16

patient from the Royal Marsden Hospital and I were there to give the patients' point of view. On 10th, Geoff and I attended the Faraday lecture at Manchester Free Trade Hall. In 1979 it was given by EMI and covered the period from the discovery of X rays to the invention of Computerised Tomography.

And so the hectic pace of life continued. I drove myself to a variety of functions in the North West. These included another visit to Rossendale and to the Pan Book Conference in Chester. The latter had a happily significant result for one of their representatives, but more of that later. Then the calendar informed me that it was May and when the pace showed no sign of slackening, the family complained that I was driving myself into the ground.

'Why d'you take so much on?'

'Because if people are supporting something I started then I feel I have a responsibility to attend the events they organise, if I possibly can.'

Yet it did mean quite a sacrifice of family life – and who knew how much of that was left to me?

For example: our daughter Helen, our son-in-law Gerard and our baby grand-daughter lived in a small flat in Toxteth, Liverpool. Gerard had to be away overnight on a field trip in connection with his degree studies at Liverpool University. Helen took the opportunity to pay us a brief visit, arriving in Preston in time for Geoff to meet her train at 5 p.m. At 8 p.m. I was due at the Highbury Club in Fleetwood. Much as I would have loved to have spent the evening cuddling my little Victoria, and chatting with my daughter, in all conscience, I *couldn't* let people down at the last minute.

As things turned out, it proved to be one of the happiest and most hilarious nights of the scanner trail.

The club room was packed with about three hundred people and the warmth of their welcome included a standing ovation. A lot of the men present with their wives were Fleetwood trawlermen – as hardy and generous a breed as

17

you'd find anywhere. They reminded me of the crew of the Fleetwood lifeboat, with whom, as a reporter, I'd made a trip to the Morecambe Bay lightship to deliver Christmas presents. A distance of twenty-five sea miles, it had been as calm as the proverbial mill pond as we left harbour. But in the unpredictable Irish Sea a Force 9 gale had sprung up, seemingly out of nowhere. The mast began to sway like a metronome. The little boat staggered to the crest of each mountainous wave, teetering at the top before each watery descent into the next trough sent it lurching either to port or starboard or head on into the oncoming wall of water. When we finally drew alongside the lightship, transferring from one vessel to the other for the Christmas carol service, as planned, proved to be impossible. With the boats bobbing like a couple of corks, we waited for the most advantageous moment and then the lightship crew quite literally, had their Christmas dinner, mail and presents thrown at them. For me, the trip had been a most memorable experience. I wouldn't have missed it for anything. It also gave me the greatest respect, not only for their courage, but also for the stamina of their stomachs. When you can nonchalantly eat a meat pie and down a pint of ale in those conditions . . . Yours truly was sick (just once) but nevertheless found the trip exhilarating and it left me with the greatest admiration for seafaring folk.

But back to the Highbury Club. For the first part of the evening there were several artistes to entertain us. Then somebody swiped the organist's stool, put it in the middle of the small dance floor and threw a tarpaulin over it. Next, two men staggered in with a huge orange PVC crate, out of the corner of which protruded a tail fit for a mermaid.

We were about to have a fish auction. The auctioneer and his assistant began with half a dozen pairs of kippers — several times over. Then they progressed to plaice and codling. Looking at the enormous tail, I nudged Pauline. 'What d'you suppose is on the other end of that?'

We were soon to find out. Meanwhile, everything being

18

auctioned was put into white plastic carrier bags. Then the auctioneer's assistant delved his hand into the bowels of the crate, the tail began to disappear and we watched, hypnotised as the most gigantic cod with the ugliest face you ever saw, was held aloft for display. It must have measured all of six feet or more.

'Now what am I bid for this?' asked the auctioneer.

Amid hilarious repartee and unrepeatable comments as to what he could do with it, it was sold for a fiver, far less than its commercial value. It was promptly given back. Re-auctioned, it again went for a fiver and was again given back. At the third attempt, some ladies on the other side of the little dance floor bought it for £3.50 whereupon the two men made a valiant attempt to stuff the hapless fish into a carrier bag. It was just about the ultimate in optimism and brought the house down. The ladies put the bag beneath the table at which they were sitting, but the fish began to ooze out looking for all the world like the Loch Ness monster. The men went on to auction shrimps, prawns, a couple of lobsters and other finned or shelled varieties of seafood.

On reflection, the ladies must have decided they didn't know what to do with the massive cod and gave it back. Dead though it was, the fish seemed to assume an increasingly mournful expression.

So did the auctioneer and his assistant.

They looked around the entire audience with expressions of disgust.

'We've got that bloody cod back again! And the next b. . . who gets it, can bloody well keep it!'

The assembled company, including Pauline and I were doubled up with laughter.

Eventually, some fellow gave £2.50 for it. It was enough to keep a fish and chip shop going for a week.

We went home with a cheque for over £500 for the Fund and, at long past midnight, I was gutting and washing sixteen plaice. The following day, Helen took some back to Liverpool with her and what we didn't have for dinner that evening, went into the freezer. With grand folk like that to help me, I wouldn't have missed that night in Fleetwood for anything.

In complete contrast, on 11th May 1979, Geoff and I attended the annual dinner of the Manchester Junior Chamber of Commerce and Trade, which was held at the Manchester Club. A formal yet friendly affair, I was to be presented with a portrait of myself, taken by one of the North West's leading photographers to mark my election as Mancunian of the Year. The presentation was to be made by the principal guest of honour, Sir Harold Wilson. To tell you the truth, until that evening I hadn't formed any opinion of him. I probably knew as much or as little about him as most members of the public.

President Alan Ward introduced me and I, in turn, introduced my husband. There followed informal conversation until it was time for dinner. Geoff found it fascinating to be in the company of a man who had been at the centre of national and international politics for so many years. After the meal, Sir Harold spoke for some fifteen minutes and then spent some time answering the questions put to him by members.

It was all very interesting but I have to admit that I found the second speaker more to my taste.

Peter Maloney has the reputation of being a first rate raconteur and it is a reputation which is fully justified. A former Trappist monk and a former Army parachutist, he entertained us with his native Liverpool wit, with one anecdote after another, leaving us with our ribs aching. Peter is now a college lecturer and one story in particular stays in my mind. It concerned an encounter on a London underground train. Peter was seated and strap-hanging above him was one of his former students. They greeted each other. Then:

'Hey – d'you remember that lecture you gave us on ethics?'

'Yes.'

'Well, I failed the practical.'

An encounter with another well-known Liverpool wit – my dear friend Ken Dodd, took place later in the month when, as Patron of the Fund, he came to a meeting of the Branch Committees from many parts of the North West which was held at the Christie staff club.

A couple of weeks earlier, I had telephoned him.

'Ken, you've done endless free shows to help raise money for my Appeal. How d'you feel about giving three-quarters of a million of it away?'

He whistled.

'Three-quarters of a million? Who's on the receiving end?'

'The Chairman of the Area Health Authority.'

Not only had we to provide the scanner, plus the building, which was a complete department, but we had also to guarantee the financial cost over a period of ten years. The A.H.A. were to invest the money and use it for this purpose as and when it was required. The figure arrived at was the result of amicable discussion between the Fund Treasurer and A.H.A. officials. It was another significant milestone along the scanner trail.

After the formalities were over, Ken was signing autographs. Someone remarked: 'That's b– awful writing!'

Quite unabashed, Ken retorted: 'Doctor's writing,' and handed it to the recipient with: 'Here – take two, three times a day.'

And so the weeks sped by.

I had a call from Audrey Brindle, chairman of the Wigan branch of the Fund. A mastectomy patient, Audrey was the jolliest character. In spite of her own problem and also having a mentally handicapped son to care for, she was full of fun and had an infinite capacity for making the best of things. She certainly got results. The Rector of Wigan, Malcolm Forrest, loved her dearly but described Audrey's efforts as 'organised chaos'. At the drop of a hat, she'd raised about £1,600 for the repair of his church roof, roping in everyone to help whether they had intended to or not. A devout Christian, but not in the least sanctimonious, Audrey just left her life in God's hands and got on with living. But I knew what the Rector meant.

On one occasion, I had a full day's itinerary in Wigan and had arranged to meet Audrey in a lay-by just off the M6 motorway. It was more than an hour later than the pre-arranged time when we did meet – Audrey having waited in one lay-by and I in another. Another time, due to a mix-up of dates resulting in a double booking, I arrived at a Fashion Show in Wigan after a mad dash from Rochdale, just in time to see the last model walk down the catwalk.

They say you can insult your friends but one is polite to one's enemies. If that is true, then Audrey and I were the greatest of friends. One day I had a phone call. 'Hey, you old divil! I do plenty to help you. Now I want you to do something to help me.'

'What is it?'

'I want you to crown Wigan Carnival Queen on 9th June.'

'With pleasure. That's always supposing she doesn't mind hanging around for a couple of hours whilst you and I get lost!'

'You cheeky so-and-so! *You* are notorious for getting lost on your travels. In fact it's become a standing joke with all of us on the Fund. Don't worry, I'll make sure that you are in the right place at the right time.'

'And I'll believe *that* when it happens!'

We both laughed.

What a happy day that was. Bands, fancy costumes, numerous decorated floats and the whole town *en fête*. As a member of the organising committee, Audrey was dashing in half a dozen directions at once (or so it seemed), checking that no detail had been overlooked. The Queen was crowned with all due ceremony *and* at the appointed time and the sun shone down on us all.

Then, later in the month came the blessed peace of Trearddur Bay, Anglesey. My husband describes Trearddur 'like putting on an old familiar coat – you know it is going to fit and that you'll be comfortable with it.' I know what he means. The unchanging beauty of that stretch of coastline is, in itself, a kind of security. There is continuity, too. Over almost three decades we have progressed from watching our own children toddling about on the beach to recent times when we enjoy making sand castles for our grand-daughter. For me, it is time spent with my family, and that is treasure beyond price.

3

AS PAULINE HAS so often remarked, you never know what's
going to happen next at this house.

The last weekend of July and I had driven home along the
motorways in the small hours of Sunday morning, having
attended a function some forty miles away. At 10.00 a.m.,
Geoff was getting ready to go to church. 'It's no good, love, I
just can't raise the energy this week. Say one for me when
you're there.'

When he had left the house at about twenty past ten, I
turned over in bed, enjoying that glorious euphoria between sleeping and waking. Sheer bliss . . .

Twenty minutes later, I heard the downstairs 'phone ring
like a clarion. *Oh, blast!*

I stretched out an arm, reaching for the bedside exten-
sion, groped for the receiver and gave the number.

'Is that Pat Seed?' asked a bright male voice.

'Yes.'

'Oh. I couldn't be so close to your home without contact-
ing you. I'd love to meet you and have a chat. I feel we'd
have a lot in common.'

At that moment, I hadn't the slightest inclination to have
anything in common with anybody. However, the bright
voice continued:

'My name is John Slater. I'm walking from Land's End to

24

John O'Groats in my pyjamas and bare feet, accompanied by my black Labrador dog called Guinness who is wearing purple boots'.

Guinness . . . I sat bolt upright in bed, trying to take it in. At last night's event I had drunk nothing more than bitter lemon, yet a glance in the dressing table mirror didn't do a thing to improve my morale.

I *looked* like the morning after the night before.

'Oh yes?' was all I could think of to say.

'Yes, it's quite an adventure.'

'Where are you now?'

He mentioned a small village about five miles away.

'I've stayed with some awfully nice people and they said I really ought to meet you.'

My sleepy mind struggled to cope.

'If you'd like to come and have coffee with us . . .' hoping the invitation didn't sound too unenthusiastic.

'Thank you. I'll look forward to that, but it will take me at least an hour to reach you. Remember, you don't travel so fast on bare feet.' An hour. That would give me time to make myself presentable – with a bit of luck – whip a duster round the house, etc. As a precaution, I threw a few extra spuds in the oven to cook alongside the roast.

By the time I'd done all this, Geoff returned from church. I met him at the front door.

'There's a chap coming in a minute. He's wearing pyjamas, he's barefooted and his dog has purple boots.' I giggled at my better half's expression of incredulity.

Before he had time to ask if I'd gone stark raving bonkers, I looked over his shoulder and added: 'As a matter of fact, he's just turned in at the end of the drive.'

'You've got to be joking!'

But as I called out 'Hello, John. Come on in,' he turned round and we both took stock of our visitor.

The only thing he'd forgotten to mention was the most enormous rucksack which framed his torso, his amiable face and shock of golden hair. He seemed to ooze good health

25

out of every pore. So much so, that instead of feeling one degree under, I reassessed my rating into double figures.

We all trooped into the sitting room and I served the coffee.

'What is the purpose of your walk?' I asked.

It seemed that John had a very good executive job somewhere in the south of England but had decided that he was caught up in the rat race. He had opted out and had gone to work with mentally handicapped children in Ayrshire. He had become friendly with Dr Tom McAllister of the Royal Hospital for Sick Children in Glasgow. Although he wasn't sponsored, he was doing his marathon walk to draw attention to the hospital's need for funds and his rig out was a publicity gimmick. En route, he'd met many individuals and groups of good natured folk who had subsequently forwarded money to Glasgow.

Local papers from Land's End to Lancashire had a field day and he'd had some radio and TV coverage. He also had an entertaining fund of anecdotes – enough to fill a book – and he was an excellent raconteur. By this time, we had polished off the roast and all that went with it. John opened a tin of dog food for Guinness, a beautiful, sleek, obedient creature who, as luck would have it, was just coming into season. This, of course, aroused my King Charles spaniel's amorous instincts, but Guinness wasn't interested. In any case the respective sizes of bitch and dog would have made the mating game a near impossibility. To save hassle and embarrassment the two animals spent alternate periods in the garden.

'Why purple boots? Is that part of the gimmick, too?'

No, it was no gimmick – although it helped. There was a very practical reason. John was walking on pavements and metalled roads, so that he could see where he was putting his feet.

'Grass would be more comfortable, but you can't see bits of broken glass or other hazards,' he explained. 'If I cut my feet, I've had it.' More used to bounding over grassland,

26

the purple boots of leather and corduroy were to protect Guinness's pads from hard road surface wear and tear. At roughly the half way stage of their journey, both John's feet and the dog's pads were in excellent shape.

'How do you manage practicalities such as washing clothes?'

'Oh, I do a bit of dobeying as and when I can. I manage.'

I offered John the use of my automatic washer and some time later I was pegging about seven pairs of gaily coloured pyjamas on the line. Heaven knows what the neighbours thought!

It reminded John of an incident in either Gloucester or Worcester – I forget which town – when in the early hours of the morning he had gone into an all night launderette, stripped down to his underpants and shoved everything else in one of the washers. He sat back, almost hypnotized by the machine's rotation and with Guinness flaked out at his feet, thinking he had the place to himself.

But no. In came a lady towing a shopping trolley of laundry.

'Good morning,' said John.

'Mornin'.' The lady weighed up the situation. After a lengthy, shocked silence, she eventually ventured to ask:

'Are those your underpants?'

'Yes.'

'Where are your clothes?'

'In Scotland.'

'Then what's in that washer?'

'My pyjamas.'

Convinced that she'd met with an escaped lunatic, the lady made for the door, jamming her trolley in it and spilling half her laundry on to the street in the process.

Who could blame her? Mad dogs and Englishmen might be daft enough to go out in the midday sun, as Noël Coward put it, but you don't expect to find them almost starkers in a launderette in the middle of the night.

Anecdote followed anecdote. We discussed some of the

27

places along his route, some of which we knew and some we didn't. Tea time came and went. Geoff had brought home a pile of work from the office to read, learn and inwardly digest in preparation for an important meeting later in the week. With such excellent company as a distraction, he never gave it a thought.

'Where are you going to sleep tonight?' I asked John.

'Oh, I'll probably find a barn or something. I once slept in a roadman's hut,' he told us with a wry grimace. 'It wasn't the most comfortable of places in which to doss down, but as it was pouring torrential rain, it was better than open ground.'

'We've a couple of spare bedrooms. You and Guinness can use one of those if you like. You're very welcome.' After John had a good hot soak in the bath, he and his canine companion settled down for the night.

Pauline was sitting at the desk next morning when John and Guinness made an appearance. Her face was a study. I giggled.

More conversation followed, plus a 'phone call to Dr McAllister in Glasgow. I sent the stoic traveller on his way replete with a breakfast of fruit juice, cereal, eggs, bacon and tomatoes, toast and marmalade and a huge pot of coffee.

It was almost midday.

When we had the house to ourselves, I grinned at Pauline, knowing there would be some reaction.

'Well?'

'Well – what? I always knew I worked in a mad house. Today's just another example.' Fortunately she was laughing as she said it.

'Anyhow, you can't say it's dull, can you?'

'Dull! Nothing would surprise me here. Now, d'you think we could get down to some work?' indicating the pile of letters on the desk.

Some weeks later I saw John being interviewed on TV at John O'Groats; he'd made it and I was glad.

Where life may eventually lead him is anyone's guess, but for a brief period he'd been doing his own thing and doing a bit of good for others, too. And for a few brief hours, he'd certainly enlivened the Seed household. It had been worth missing a couple of hours extra sleep, to meet the man who came for coffee.

And so July and August drifted by and each time I visited the Christie I looked anxiously at the building progress. Initially, the completion date and the arrival of the scanner were scheduled for the end of September. It is inevitable, I suppose, in an undertaking of this magnitude that there should be unforeseen snags and delays. But with nerves becoming more ragged as the publication date of my book drew nearer, plus the fact that every day of delay meant that some patients weren't getting the benefit of the scanner, for the first time since the founding of the Appeal, I 'lost my cool'.

I rang the architect, a kindly intelligent man who had always been most helpful and asked for some straight answers. It seemed they couldn't finish off until they'd got certain things finalised with EMI. I rang EMI. *They* were waiting for completion of certain parts of the building! The scanner would not arrive until November. That did it.

'For heaven's sake, get your heads together and get the darned job finished. It's going to look fine in the Press isn't it, if none of you can meet your deadlines. All the people who have raised the money are going to want to know why.'

Tony Layzell, EMI's European Marketing Director, assured me that everything possible would be done. Much later, Tony told me that the architect had said to him: 'I've just been bounced all round my office by Pat Seed. Do you know, she actually swore at me!'

I was decidedly unpopular and I didn't give a damn. The workmen went on extra time and things began to move. The final test on the scanner before it was crated for shipment in Chicago was five days continuous running. On the fifth day, it broke down. The fault was rectified and there began another five days of continuous running.

Would it ever arrive?

It would be a couple of years later when Tony told me the following story.

Knowing of my poor prognosis he had asked my consultant how he accounted for the fact that I was still alive two and a half years later. My consultant thought for a moment and then replied:

'I don't know. I don't think cancer stood much of a chance against Pat – any more than the rest of us!'

I had hooted with laughter.

'Oh, Tony! You make me sound an absolute martinet!'

'Don't worry, Pat. They are all very fond of you. It's just that when you get that certain gleam in your eyes, they do wonder what's coming next. I know the feeling,' he grinned.

At a Central Committee meeting, Sir William Downward, Lord Lieutenant of Greater Manchester and our chairman, said that he thought that the Royal opening of the department might probably take place in December or early in the new year. Seeing a red velvet suit which I thought might do for the occasion, I bought it. But it wasn't destined to be worn at the Royal opening.

And then came the day, the thought of which had given me the collywobbles all year – 11th October and the publication of *One Day At a Time*.

Why should I feel like this? As a journalist, seeing my reports in print had long ceased to have novelty. But a journalist is the intermediary between the event and the reader. The aim is to be as factually correct as possible, whether we are reporting what we call 'hard news' or writing a feature about a person or topic of current interest. The difference was that the book was *me*, my story.

Before having cancer I had lived happily on my own little cabbage patch, running my home and following the profession I loved. Inevitably, the Appeal Fund had thrust me before the eyes of the public through TV, radio and news-paper coverage of its progress. Now, my version of the incredible events of the last two and a half years was to make my life an open book. It turned out to be one of the most hectic, hardworking periods of my life.

The build up began a couple of weeks before publication with interviews by various newspaper colleagues and radio interviews. I seemed to be up and down the Inter-city line to London like a yo-yo. Either Marie, my dear friend and district nurse or Pauline accompanied me, for Geoff will not let me be away from home overnight on my own, in case I am taken ill and need help. On one of these trips, Marie and I had dinner with another good friend, Jean Rook. Marie, who has a zany sense of humour (which is why we get on so well) and a fund of unprintable anecdotes, had Jean in stitches, prompting her to say to me:

'They ought to put her on the telly and just let her run on until she dries up.' I think I said that no programme would be long enough. In our turn, Marie and I enjoyed a series of anecdotes à la Rook – and there's only one Jean Rook. She adheres strictly to the truth and, more often than not, writes what many people are thinking but would be afraid to say. A courageous journalist, a sincere, down-to-earth Yorkshire-woman and a good friend. The following day I had a series of interviews at radio stations in London and I had not realised that there were so many. Marie said that she felt like Alice in Wonderland. We began early in the morning and finished at nine at night, with just a twenty minute break for lunch. Programmes or recordings included the BBC World Service and overseas programmes as well as local BBC and commercial stations. The whole day seemed to be spent wending our way through London's traffic; in and out of taxis; up elevators and into studios. A couple of days later, there were interviews for Radio Carlisle and Radio Ulster and then, back to London yet again, this time for Russell Harty's Midweek programme. Back home in time for tea and an early night, for the following day I had the first of my book signing sessions, appropriately, in Garstang, where the story had begun.

In between the morning and afternoon signings, I met Mrs. Margaret Thatcher. The Conservative Party Conference was taking place at Blackpool and our M.P. Sir Walter Clegg had arranged for us to meet. Brief though the audience was, I found the Prime Minister to be a woman of utmost charm and femininity and with a warmth of personality. Of her sincerity and her concern for Britain there is no shadow of doubt. More signing sessions followed in the ensuing days and on 16th I did a lunchtime signing in Kendal Milne, Manchester, where Geoff and I were entertained to lunch; then, on to Menzies bookshop in Salford before making a mad dash by car to Piccadilly station to catch a train to Coventry in order to keep a very special date.

At the Women of the Year Luncheon at the Savoy Hotel, London in September 1978, H.R.H. The Duchess of Kent had expressed an interest in the Fund and had graciously offered her help. Through the Combined Charities Commission, she had intended to hold an event in March, but her illness had meant that it had to be postponed. Now the Duchess was to attend a Royal Gala Performance in the Coventry Theatre. A star studded variety programme, the Three Degrees topped the bill and at the end of the evening, Her Royal Highness presented me with a very substantial cheque for the Fund. Our worry had been whether or not we would get to the theatre on time. We had to change trains at Birmingham and found that the city was in the throes of a bus strike. It seemed as if the entire commuter population had taken to the train. The only space Geoff and I could find on the Coventry train, was the guard's van. The guard kindly offered me his swivel seat which I thankfully accepted. The train stopped at every little station between Birmingham and Coventry. The journey seemed endless and each time the train negotiated a bend in the track, yours truly nearly went into orbit. We arrived at our hotel, had a quick cup of tea and a sandwich, spruced ourselves with a quick wash and change and just scraped into the theatre before Her Royal Highness arrived.

We were back in Manchester the next day for a lunchtime signing and during the week that followed there were similar sessions in various north west towns. By now, I was so tired I didn't know whether I was on my head or my heels. I was thankful that my name has only seven letters. After all, I could have been stuck with a name such as Henrietta Winterbottom – not that there's anything wrong with the name. It just takes longer to write.

And so the hectic month progressed and on 26th I attended a quite different, but no less enjoyable variety concert. It was organised by the staff of Blackburn Fire Station.

Even though I was the principal guest and consequently 'on view' I regarded it as a night off, after the hectic pace of the past few weeks.

A great deal of preparation had gone into that event. I find it most moving to see the lengths to which people go in support of the Fund. In this case, all the fire tenders had been parked in the yard and the huge garage converted into a concert hall, with a stage at one end and with greenery decorating the walls. As on so many other occasions, the artistes gave their performances for free. But before the concert got under way, we were warned that should there be a fire, the stage amplification would be switched off whilst firemen received their instructions over the tannoy.

Everything was fine until about a third of the way through the evening. A comedian had just got to the punch line of a long story when his microphone went dead. Over the tannoy came a sepulchral voice:

'Will firemen Smith, Jones and Brown report to the fire tender number one. There is a chip pan fire at . . .'

The attention of the entire audience was riveted on Messrs Smith, Jones and Brown as they grabbed their gear and with a speed which would have done credit to Sebastian Coe, sprinted into the yard and fire tender number one hurtled off into the night with blue light flashing and siren wailing. By the time his microphone was 'live' again, the comedian had not only forgotten his punch line, but which joke he'd been telling us.

There were three fires in Blackburn that night. It must have been disconcerting for the artistes, but they all took it in good part. As for the audience, most of them were firemen or their families. For them, it was just one of the penalties of the job and it didn't seem to stop anyone enjoying themselves, which is more than can be said for the poor folks whose properties were on fire.

As I write about occasions such as this, I am very conscious of those I do not mention, put on by people equally as generous and warm hearted. To attempt to record every function, every event would result in a catalogue of unmanageable proportions. But, dear reader, be of no doubt whatever, how much I appreciate the efforts people have made – and still are making – to help keep the Christie abreast of the latest technology.

It reminds me of that wartime slogan 'give us the tools and we'll finish the job'. Although much valuable progress has been made in recent years in the fight against the many forms of cancer, there is still a long way to go. As research progresses, so does technology. It must be frustrating beyond measure for doctors experienced and brilliant in the field of cancer medicine, to know that there are items of equipment which might help to save or prolong life – if only they could afford to buy them out of NHS funds. Such is the essence of my Fund and most people appreciate my slogan: 'The life you help to save could be yours.' For there is hardly a family in the land, rich or poor, who hasn't lost a relative or a friend with this scourge of mankind.

4

A FEW DAYS rest and then Pauline and I were off again, this time to Yorkshire. The 31st October was Hallowe'en, just the night to stay at the ancient Silent Inn, near the Brontë village of Haworth. It even had a ghost! We were to attend two literary dinners and a literary lunch at three different places, a bi-monthly event organised by the *Yorkshire Ridings* magazine and the *Lancashire Magazine*. The after dinner speakers were Rona Randall, author of some fifty novels; Roger Mason, author of *Granny's Village* whose second book *The Great Skipton Show* had just been published, plus yours truly – the novice. Both Roger and I are Heinemann authors and Steven Williams, their publicity manager was there to give us moral support or any assistance that we might need. Except for Roger and his wife whom we were to meet later, at the first rendezvous, we arrived at the Silent Inn at about five o'clock. We waited with interest for Rona to arrive, for I had read and enjoyed many of her books. But by seven o'clock, when we were due to leave for an hotel in Bingley, there was no sign of her. Eventually, Winston Halstead and Joan Laprell, the editor and assistant editor of *Yorkshire Ridings* magazine, decided we had better be moving. As we left the Inn to walk across the car park, a taxi swept into the drive, came to a halt and out stepped a

35

diminutive blonde in a full length mink coat. Her first words were: 'I've had a dreadful journey. I *must* have a bath and freshen up before I do *anything*'.

Tactfully, I suggested that we go on ahead and 'hold the fort' until she arrived at the Bingley hotel. Rona was accompanied by a young American girl, a representative of her publishing company.

It was agreed that at the three events we would take it in turn to be first, second or third speaker, and we were advised to restrict our talks to fifteen minutes each. At Bingley, I was to start the ball rolling and, being Hallowe'en, I only briefly mentioned my book, for I couldn't resist regaling the audience with ghostly anecdotes, including the Lancashire Witches. I recalled the time when we had taken our Vancouver friends, Noel and Kay Beaumont on a tour of Pendle witch country. The party had included my parents and our children so two cars had been necessary. With Geoff driving his former wartime pilot and the other menfolk, I followed behind with the females of the party crammed into the car I then had – an old red banger of a mini.

Driving that car was an adventure in that one never knew what would go wrong next. We toured most of the villages mentioned in Robert Neil's *Mist Over Pendle* and as we started the return journey, we were passing beneath the shadow of Pendle Hill, which always manages to look forbidding, no matter what time of the year it is or what the weather might be. It was at this point that Kay, in her Canadian accent said:

'Say, are there still witches around here?'

I laughed. 'No. Not these days, thank goodness.'

About fifty yards further on, there was an ominous clang under the bonnet of the mini and it came to a grinding halt. We could see Geoff's car disappearing round a corner ahead of us. By this time, it was getting dark and had started to rain. We sat there, waiting to be missed and it seemed an eternity before Geoff returned to look for us. At a nearby farm he was given a length of stout rope (for towing) and we began a long slow crawl back to Garstang, where we thankfully left the mini at a local garage. It cost just £13 to have the fault put right. No Lancashire witches? I'll never scoff at them again.

Then it was Roger's turn. I cannot remember a great deal of what he said, for the microphone kept falling off its stand at regular intervals. It happened so many times that I felt obliged to inform the company that the Lancashire witches did not extend their activities to Yorkshire – I hoped! Rona then gave a most interesting account of her work, her method of writing, her early years as an author, but like Roger and me she over ran her allotted time. As Winston told the three of us later, 'When you are talking, you are not selling books.'

Back at the Silent Inn, we found, much to Pauline's relief, that Steven had been allocated the room supposedly haunted by a little serving maid of several centuries ago who rattled her keys. The following morning he told us that he had neither seen nor heard anything of her. In fact, he'd slept like a top. I chided him that, coming from a famous publishing house, the least he could have done was to have borrowed a bag of flour from our host and come downstairs with hair supposedly turned white overnight.

'But on second thoughts, you would sleep peacefully. It was well after midnight when we all went to bed and by that time it would be All Saints Day. No self respecting ghost would haunt on *that* day.'

The next lunchtime saw us all at an old hall at Luddenden near Halifax. This time, my talk did not over run and I took pleasure in telling this Yorkshire audience of the Duchess of Kent's part in the Appeal; how much I was indebted to her and how very proud of her they must be. I was left in no doubt of the affection of these good Yorkshire folk for 'their' member of the Royal Family.

Rona had been primed by her young American girl on what she should say and what she shouldn't say. She found it inhibiting, to say the least, and in an effort to comply, again over ran her time.

It was at this venue that I met again the Pan representative who had attended the Chester meeting earlier in the year. He said to me:

'I've come to see you to say "thank you" Pat.'

Somewhat bewildered, I asked him what on earth he had to thank me for.

It was then that he explained that after listening to me at the Chester meeting, he had gone home and asked his wife if she had had the cervical smear test. Apparently she had not had this simple check up and he had advised his good lady that it was a sensible thing to do. A day or two later, she had her test which proved positive, showing the early warning signs of cancer of the neck of the womb. Her problem had been dealt with, the trouble arrested and she was now fit and well. The Pan representative was well aware that his wife could have been in serious trouble had she not taken this simple precaution.

'But for hearing what you had to say to us at Chester it would never have occurred to either of us and I just wanted you to know how grateful we both feel.'

Oh, that all women would follow suit. So much misery and distress could be avoided.

After lunch we were all to make our way to an hotel in Gisburn, Lancashire for the final dinner. But as Pauline and I headed for my car, we noticed that Steven had left in search of some more of Roger's books. Joan and Winston's car was piled high with books so that they had no spare seat; Miss America had departed for London, leaving Rona to 'go it alone'. So we offered Rona a seat in my car and as we drove through the lovely autumn countryside of West Yorkshire and East Lancashire we learned that 'I've had a dreadful journey' was just about the understatement of the year. Rona had left her home in Hayward's Heath, Sussex at some unearthly hour of the morning and had spent a cold and miserable time waiting for 'Miss America' who had turned up two hours late at King's Cross station. They had taken the Leeds train instead of the Bradford train and on arrival, had waited over half an hour in a taxi queue. The driver of the taxi hadn't heard of the Silent Inn and Rona had more or less done the grand tour of Yorkshire before she finally reached her destination. No wonder she was fed up.

Rona is a woman with a lively sense of fun which, thank goodness, had only temporarily deserted her. On the journey, we did our best to restore her morale. We arrived at the Gisburn hotel in plenty of time for a rest before the final event. Even then, the capricious fate which had dogged her hadn't finished. Finding it impossible to get water to run into the bath, she summoned help and a man (who later had the role of wine waiter at dinner) provided a temporary solution by fixing a hosepipe to the washbasin tap, with the other end of it draped over the side of the bath. This, Pauline and I learned when we all met for pre-dinner drinks. Just as the gin and tonics were served Winston came into the bar.

His opening gambit was; 'Now Rona, I'm going to be very strict with you,' (about the length of her speech) whereupon Rona put a wisp of a handkerchief to her lips and rushed from the room.

Pauline and I looked at each other.

'D'you think I had better go after her?' asked my soft hearted secretary.

'Yes – and take that gin and tonic with you.'

I grinned at Winston, who was really a charming host and did his best to make things easy for us.

'You may be lucky if you have three speakers tonight. You might only have two. You know, Rona hasn't had an easy time of it, one way and another.'

Meanwhile, Pauline found Rona sitting on a chair outside her room. She had been too upset to remember to collect her key from reception. Pauline found a few words of comfort and then added:

'You know, when things go wrong for Pat and me on the

Appeal, we have a good moan; then we say "sod it!", have a good laugh and then get on with the job.'

Neither Pauline or I are prone to using bad language. There are far more effective adjectives than 'bloody' and so on. But at times of utter frustration, those two words do relieve the situation, as I believe even Angela Rippon admits.

Rona looked at Pauline with her wide blue eyes. Then she said firmly: 'Sod it!' – and burst out laughing. Eventually, they both came downstairs. I said that with more than fifty books under her belt, she was entitled to say what she liked. 'Give your talk *your* way, Rona. Just be yourself and re- member that there are two Lancashire lasses rooting for you.'

Her speech that evening was the best of the lot – witty, engaging and perfectly natural. As for me, I found it an odd experience to see in the audience some of the people mentioned in my book. People like Jack and Edith Marsden, the former Mayor and Mayoress of South Ribble, who had supported the Fund so loyally. Also Maxine Hukin of Barnoldswick, another good supporter who, when I was awarded the MBE had written to say that the letters stood for 'many blessings eternally'.

Rona left at some unearthly hour for Yeadon, to catch a plane to Heathrow. She'd been awake half the night. Her computerised calculator – cum – clock with an alarm had sounded on the hour, every hour throughout the night and she was damned if she could figure out how to switch the thing off! On her return home she wrote us a highly amusing letter which had Pauline and me laughing. We still keep in touch with Rona and always enjoy the occasions when we meet.

For Pauline and me the trip had been one of the happiest experiences to date. We were back in Garstang for Friday lunchtime and next day I went to a service in Chester Cathedral. It was dedicated to those concerned with cancer, both those who suffered and those whose work is the care of cancer patients. Attending it were many of my friends from Farndon, a small village a few miles outside the ancient city, where the entire population had held a series of efforts and raised about £2,000 for the Fund.

After the Oncology Conference at Oxford, I had been invited to attend a similar conference of the Welsh Branch of the Royal College of Nursing at Velindre Hospital, Cardiff. Marie accompanied me on this trip, but before we left Preston station a wonderful thing happened. My dear friend and fellow journalist, Tess Pickford, had just got off the London train. We fell into each others' arms and both of us cried. She had left Garstang to spend two years doing Voluntary Service Overseas in the Solomon Islands, running a school for trainee journalists. In September 1977 our leave taking had been a sad affair, for neither expected to see the other again. With my poor prognosis, we had thought it to be the final 'goodbye'. Yet, here I was, still around to see her return home at the end of her two year stint. Oh, God was good. He was good, indeed. Promising to get together as soon as we could, I travelled down to Cardiff on cloud nine and with a thankful heart. I looked forward to more of our good times together, for Tess has a dry wit and a capacity for making the most unlikely or outlandish undertaking seem perfectly feasible. I would be able to enjoy her company until those itchy feet of hers sent her haring off again to some other far-flung part of the globe.

Marie and I arrived in Cardiff on the Tuesday evening and the Wednesday morning conference was very worthwhile. We caught an afternoon train back to Preston, changing at Crewe and arriving home at about 10 p.m.

There were about a dozen telephone messages on the pad, but I didn't even attempt to deal with them. I was far too tired and my brain was addled. As I tottered up to bed I thought to myself, 'This is how boxers must feel when they're punch drunk' and wondered for how much longer I could keep up the pace at which I was living. Sick woman? I didn't have the time to think whether I was sick or not!

41

On 28th November, in company with five distinguished people, I received an Honorary Fellowship of Manchester Polytechnic. The other recipients were Dame Kathleen Ollerenshaw, Group Captain Leonard Cheshire, Mr Bobby Charlton, Mr Ralph Ruddock and Mr Simon Goldstone. I had been asked to give the speech of reply on behalf of the honorands.

The previous evening Geoff and I were going out for a meal with friends whom we were due to meet at eight o'clock. I made a point of getting myself ready early so that I could draft my speech. Until now I had never used a written speech, preferring to talk spontaneously to people. But sitting there with pad and pen, I'd get half a sentence written and the 'phone would ring. In the next hour, it rang nine times, so that in the end, I gave up trying to get my speech down on paper. Although I knew what I wanted to say, I would have to deliver it my usual way, putting my thoughts into words as I went along. I suppose it was the best way, really. If you try to be pretentious, or anything other than what you are, you generally come a cropper. With a sheaf of notes, maybe nervousness would have made me drop them all over the floor. I was concerned that I did not let down the other people on behalf of whom I would be speaking.

After lunch the conferment ceremony was held and each of us in turn was presented to the Director, Sir Alec Smith, by one of the Polytechnic's lecturers. Miss Gisella Bergman kindly presented me. All of us wore gowns and mortar boards. As we were received, Sir Alec invested each of us with the orange and black hood, denoting our new status. In my speech of reply, I commented on the diversity of talents of the other five honorands and said that to use one's talents for one's own satisfaction gave fulfilment; when those talents were used for the benefit of other people, therein lay the true fulfilment. I ended by thanking Sir Alec and Manchester Polytechnic for the honour they paid us.

Rooms had been booked for us at the Midland Hotel, to

which we retired for a rest before the dinner at the Polytechnic that evening. As Group Captain Cheshire and my husband and I were stepping into the car which was to take us to the dinner, my 'This Is Your Life' programme went on the screen. It had been recorded at the New Drury Lane Theatre just a week previously. Geoff and I couldn't watch it, being otherwise engaged, but friends later told me that Garstang was like a ghost town for that half hour, with most of the local population glued to their TV sets. Transmission was impaired somewhat in the North West of England and for just about the most unlikely reason you could think of. A recent sand storm in the Sahara Desert had blown tons of fine sand up into the atmosphere. By some freak of nature, the elements had chosen that evening to shower it on the North West. In the streets, parked cars were covered with layers of sand. The following morning, newspapers carried the story, for it was the kind of happening that probably won't occur again in a thousand years. Now I ask you, who else's programme would *that* happen to?

Dinner at the Polytechnic was cooked and served in impeccable style by the catering students. It was indeed, cuisine par excellence. Each honorand was also given a silver paper knife, individually designed by one of the students. By coincidence, the young lady who designed mine came from Farndon, the village whose efforts had raised so much money for my Fund.

And then came the event for which so many of us had worked and waited. On 29th, the scanner arrived at the Christie. On 30th, we had a Central Committee meeting and we got through the agenda as quickly as we could, so that we could all go downstairs to the new department to see the new arrival. Our baby had come home. Admittedly, it was not yet dressed in its Sunday best; there were packing cases all over the place and like some gigantic jigsaw puzzle, it would take time to assemble. In charge of this mammoth task was EMI engineer Mr Peter Clarke.

Excited and impatient as ever, I asked, how long it would

be before it went into action. I was told that assembly and thorough testing would take some six to seven weeks before it was ready to scan the first patients. That figured. But at last, the Christie *did have a scanner* and what is more, the finest and most advanced scanner in Europe.

He began his journey outside the Atomic Energy Authority premises at Risley in October 1979. Just a man and a bike. Ten days later, Ian Marshall had visited every atomic energy station in Britain supported by sponsors galore.

At Risley and Culcheth, the staff were raising money for the Pat Seed Appeal Fund, while staff at other stations, from Dounreay to Winfrith used Ian's mammoth ride to raise money for their own nominated charities. In total, over £3,600 was raised for seven different causes. On 5th December, I visited Risley to receive from Ian a cheque for £1,850. Later, some more sponsor money came in, bringing his total to over £1,900. Now *how* do you find words that are adequate enough to convey your appreciation of an effort like this? There just aren't any. But one does one's best, and at the buffet lunch provided by the Authority, I was glad to meet the staff who had supported his effort so enthusiastically.

And so 1979 drew to a close. For someone under a 'death sentence' I was doing an awful lot of living. The pace had been so drastically hectic that for most of the time I just didn't think how I was; there was so much to do. No time to spare to wallow in self pity or wonder what tomorrow might bring – it was there, in the diary, a job to do, marked out for me day by day. Only the Almighty knew how long I could keep it up. I was content to leave it at that. Our family Christmas was a happy one and I gave thanks that I was still able to share it with them.

44

5

1980 . . . AND THE FIRST day of this New Year was the third anniversary of the day I don't remember. I had spent New Year's Eve 1976 on the operating table at the Christie. I have no recollection of Christmas 1976 and the first few days of '77 are just a hazy memory of pain, discomfort and unutterable weariness. But God had other things in mind for me and had directed my feet along an entirely different route from that with which I was familiar. That He was walking it alongside of me I had no doubt, for how else could I explain where the will power, the stamina and the endurance came from?

I will never forget, even if I were to live to be a hundred, a day at the hospital in late January, when Dr Eddleston, Director of Diagnostic Radiology showed me the first scan pictures produced by *our* scanner. During the course of the Appeal, we had worn out two copies of EMI's publicity film 'The Scanner Story' which featured an earlier model. The clarity and definition of the pictures produced by the 7070 model were astounding. And to see on each one, the words 'Christie, Manchester, U.K.' really put stars in my eyes, thankfulness in my heart and an outsized lump in my throat. We'd done it! We'd actually done it – and in less than three years, for I had begun the Fund on 15th March 1977.

I thought with affection of the patients in the Christie.

How well I understood their fears and anxieties. For many of them, the scanner would offer new hope, which was far more important than having confounded the sceptics who, in the early days had said it couldn't be done. Now, it was *there*, a highly sophisticated almost miraculous technology.

For radiologists and radiotherapists it was to prove invaluable, for it yielded patient information that could be obtained by no other means. It showed more detail than could be seen by the naked eye during surgery. With it went a treatment planning system which achieved in seconds, calculations which would have taken physicists many hours. The result was an individual, tailor-made plan of treatment and with a hitherto unattainable exactitude.

But horizons were widening. At the turn of the year, more than 75,000 paperback copies of *One Day At a Time* had been sold. I received many letters from people who had found it of comfort. Others told me that they'd had difficulty seeing the print, for they'd been laughing on one page and crying on the next.

Many people added, 'Do tell us what happened next. Surely it didn't end when you laid the foundation stone?'

In the hamlet of Crowthorne, Berkshire, cancer patient Ken Thomas had been given six months to live. He determined to buy a box of cigars, a bottle of brandy and read all the books he'd never found time to read in his busy life as a schoolmaster or in his earlier years as an actor. Then his wife, Polly, bought him a copy of my book. He read it and it changed his way of life, for he decided that the hospital at which he was receiving treatment should also have a scanner. We had many telephone conversations, endless question and answer sessions and at the beginning of 1980, Ken launched his appeal with the full approval of the consultants at the Royal Berkshire Hospital, Reading. Like me, Ken was to find that he had never worked harder in his life. He was indefatigable. He cajoled, pleaded, bullied, implored and persuaded until he had an ever-increasing team of dedicated helpers around him. I promised to visit him later in the year but, meanwhile, there was other travelling to be done.

My friend, Audrey Brindle had not been well. She had another spell in hospital and was now home again. We had several chats on the phone during her stay in hospital and also when she came home. Always cheerful, always 'playing down' her situation, one day she rang me and said quietly: 'Pat, will you come to see me?' It was 3rd February.

'Audrey, love, of course I will. I'm off to Northern Ireland in the morning but I'll be home again on the 11th. I'll come to see you on the 12th.'

In the previous autumn we had visitors from Ireland at the Christie who were interested in starting an Appeal for Montgomery House, Belvoir Hospital the Province's cancer treatment centre. They had asked me to spend a few days in Northern Ireland to help them launch their Fund.

To say that family and friends had misgivings about my visit is no more than the truth. Everyone knows of the 'troubles' in the Province. But my argument was that I had no axes to grind – a cancer patient was a cancer patient, whether they lived in Ipswich, India or Ireland. Cancer was a scourge of humanity and in the name of humanity, I would go. I would not allow Pauline or Marie to come with me on this trip, for both of them had children not yet independent.

Therefore, with my pal Tess Pickford – the pair of us grandmothers – I crossed the Irish Sea, arriving in Belfast early in the evening of 4th February.

You may wonder why my husband didn't accompany me. The plain fact is, Geoff has a certain amount of annual leave. He cannot just 'take off' at the drop of a hat. As the 'year' ends on 31st March, he would have very little left. Also, he has his responsibilities and I have mine, although my activities for the Appeal have meant that my work as a journalist is practically non-existent and with a subsequent loss of income. However, there are more important things in this life than money – life itself for instance. Nevertheless,

47

someone has to 'keep our house door open'; it would be wrong and entirely unfair to expect my husband to cope with a highly responsible profession and to dash about here, there and everywhere with me. If I *had* to be away from home overnight, he had more peace of mind knowing that one of my friends was with me.

Tess and I stayed that first night at a hotel just outside Belfast and the next morning we went to Montgomery House at Belvoir Hospital to meet radiologist Dr. Geoffrey Moore, Senior Nursing Officer Mrs Winifred Tate and the Chairman of the Eastern Health Board, Sir Thomas Brown. We were made very welcome and our conversations were mostly 'scanner talk'. I gave as much information as I could and told them, in the light of my own experiences, some of the problems they may encounter and some of the pitfalls to be avoided. I think they found the exchange of views useful.

Then I visited some of the wards, chatting to patients. It was when I was in conversation with the mother of a tiny girl who was a cancer patient that BBC TV Northern Ireland came along to film a sequence for that evening's programme. In the evening we were at Ulster TV studios where I was interviewed by Gloria Hunniford. I had already agreed to be a Patron of the Appeal but I felt they also needed some Irish Patrons. Before we went on the air I asked Gloria, who of course is known all over the Province, if she would give her patronage. To this she agreed and we were able to bring it into the interview. From the studios, Tess and I were driven to an hotel in County Tyrone where we stayed for the rest of our visit.

I rang Geoff that evening, as I always do when I am away from home, just to let him know that all was well. He said that he had some sad news for me. In the early afternoon, my friend Audrey had passed away, peacefully and without pain. Her vicar, the Rev Malcolm Forrest, had given her Holy Communion just an hour before she died. I was stunned. I had promised to go to see her on my return from Ireland. Now it was too late.

48

I sat on the bed in that hotel room and cried, thinking of the gap she would leave in so many people's lives, for to know her was to love her. I thought of her family and, selfishly, thought of myself. How I would miss her affectionate bullying and teasing. My hosts asked me if I would prefer to go home. A vision of Audrey's jolly face passed before my eyes and it was as if I could almost hear her saying: 'Don't be daft, lass. What've you come to Ireland for? To help cancer patients like me! You've got a job to do – so get on and do it!'

To my hosts, 'It would be the last thing Audrey would want me to do. No, we carry out all the arrangements as planned.'

With committee member Margaret McCarroll, I went to a small neat home in the village of Fintona to meet her sister. Vonny Rafferty was bedridden and on heroin to keep her as pain free as possible. With her spirit undaunted, this young mother was in the final stages of her disease and her days were numbered. Vonny's efforts had been the first in Northern Ireland to raise money for a scanner. I would like to think that when her dream becomes a reality, Vonny's name will be remembered. We had a long talk, about life and about death which neither of us feared as we both had a strong Faith.

What worried me was that the Appeal needed some famous Irish names to be identified with it. Who more famous than Olympic Pentathlon Gold Medalist, Mary Peters? I telephoned her and explained. Her response was immediate and affirmative. Having lost near and dear ones with cancer she knew the problem only too well. The following day at the Mary Peters Sports Stadium just outside Belfast, groups of young people were doing a sponsored run around the track, which is set in a natural amphitheatre. Mary postponed an engagement long enough to come to the stadium and run the first lap with them. I, who find standing for any length of time an exhausting business, took pleasure in watching the supple grace with which this

49

great athlete moved. It reminded me of the time I had been to Southport to see Red Rum, the triple Grand National winner. Here was the same majesty of movement and controlled power. Perfection in any form is a privilege to see.

Wherever we went, Tess and I were welcomed with Irish charm and hospitality. If we had eaten everything that was offered to us, I know I would have come home at least a stone heavier. Tess, long and lanky, can eat like a stevedore without putting on an ounce.

She also had more time for observation than I. She remarked that it surprised her how many people recognised me and how genuinely appreciative they were that I was in Ireland. Very conscious of the 'troubles' in their beautiful country, ordinary Irish people of all denominations told us how much they deplored the present state of affairs.

'Do tell people, when you go back to England, that we are not *all* trouble makers,' was said to us over and over again.

One of the happiest memories is of our last evening in Northern Ireland. First, we went to Londonderry Guild Hall where a concert was to take place. We met the Mayor and several council members and some of the artistes. On Sunday evenings at home, Geoff and I often listen to the programme 'Your Hundred Best Tunes', the signature tune of which is the Londonderry Air. I never expected that one day, I should find myself here, in this beautiful place from which so many Irish people left to find a new life on the other side of the Atlantic.

'I wish someone would sing it for me,' I said.

'I will,' said a lovely Irish lady.

After I had told the large audience – some were standing, others sitting on the stairs in the great hall – of the scanner and of the task which lay ahead of them, Maureen Hegarty sang the Danny Boy lyrics to the plaintive haunting melody, supposedly written by a fairy. Her pure voice soared and you could have heard a pin drop. What a marvellous memory of Ireland for me, born on St Patrick's Day, to take home with me. Later, Maureen sent me a recording on cassette and I sent her a signed copy of my book. We drove back from Londonderry, through Strabane to Omagh in torrential rain to a concert at the Knock-na-Mo Hotel and here again, the room was full to overflowing. It was at this final venue that I was presented with a tiny gold leprechaun sitting on a toadstool for my charm bracelet and Tess was given a handsome pen. I had already been given two beautiful Belleek vases and a Tyrone crystal vase inscribed 'Pat Seed. Northern Ireland 1980.'

At some time during our visit, Tess had sauntered down to the nearest Army barracks to tell them who we were, why we were in N. Ireland (they probably knew already, but it was a matter of courtesy) and to leave a letter asking the G.O.C. Northern Ireland if H.M. Forces stationed in the Province might help with some fund-raising for the scanner. To this request I later received a letter saying that they would be happy to contribute and a year or so later I learned from the committee that the contribution from H.M. Forces had been invaluable. I was also told that, as a result of my visit, fund raising groups had been formed in many places and that over £100,000 had come in via Ulster Television after the interview with Gloria Hunniford.

When a committee member gave me a cheque for just over a hundred pounds to cover our expenses, I took great delight in scribbling over it, to cancel it. 'I think we'll let "This Is Your Life" pay for this,' I said, with a twinkle in my eyes. (My fee was £100) 'After all, Eamonn's Irish, isn't he?'

And so we left a beautiful land and some of the most attractive, hospitable people it has ever been my pleasure to meet. We left them with the slogan: 'Unite – to Fight Cancer' – the battle which confronts the whole human race.

We flew into Manchester Airport in time to drive up the M6 motorway to Wigan Parish Church to attend Audrey's funeral. Although it was a sad homecoming, the service was both comforting and uplifting. I felt that I had Audrey's approval and her love. In this life or the next, she will always be my beloved friend.

At the Christie plans were in progress for the official opening of the new department. It was to be named The Pat Seed Building. When the matter had been discussed at our Central Committee, I had put forward the name: The North West Department of Computerised Tomography, but the other members of the committee insisted that my name should be included and I was outvoted.

As the reader may have gathered, I am very sensitive to atmosphere. Standing in the reception area one day, I looked at the magnolia walls and soft green carpet and quietly reflected on the events of the last three years; all the efforts by so very many people which had made the whole thing possible. Love and a caring society had built this place. It seemed to permeate the walls and fabric of the building. The faces of some of the thousands of people who had helped, flitted across my mind, recalling the laughter, the hard work, the good nature I had encountered. It seemed as though all of these people had left a little of themselves here, to help others. God bless them all. I gave thanks for having been privileged to be a part of it all. And the lesson to be learned? That when the good side of human nature surfaces, there is so much that mankind can achieve. How sad it is that human beings spend so much time falling out with each other. Either on an individual basis or on national levels it is so *negative* when so many people in this world so desperately need a kindly word and some practical, positive help.

Her Royal Highness the Duchess of Kent had graciously agreed to open the new department on 24th April. When it comes to entertaining a member of the Royal Family, it is not Pat Seed, not the doctors of the Christie, but the Area

Health Authority who are the hosts and who are responsible for the arrangements. It has to be remembered that this large busy hospital is just not geared to entertaining large numbers of people. The largest room available on the premises was the refectory, the staff dining room. Nurses and administration staff good naturedly agreed to eat on the wards or in local pubs and restaurants that day, so that we could have the use of it. A buffet lunch was planned and I believe there had been talk of bringing in outside caterers, but the Christie catering staff had offered to make it. On the actual day, that buffet was a sight to behold. You couldn't have found a more attractive or colourful array of food set out at the Dorchester or the Savoy. The food at the Christie is always good, which is an achievement in itself when they budget for 350 patients, plus some 200 staff each day. On 24th April, they surpassed themselves.

Regrettably, the limited space meant that only one member from each branch of my Fund could be invited, to represent them all, even though 'officialdom' had been kept to a minimum. I left it to each local committee to decide which member would be their representative. Fortunately, with the exception of one committee, which promptly resigned, they all understood. To accommodate everyone would have needed a venue the size of the Albert Hall.

It is usual on such occasions for a child to present a Royal lady with flowers. There was no doubt in my mind who that child should be. No, not my little grand-daughter, much as she would have loved to do it. But more of that later.

There was the usual feminine problem of what to wear for the occasion. What would the Duchess be wearing? I would hate my outfit to clash with hers. Finally, I settled for the palest of green, a Berkertex dress with a pleated skirt and a lace bolero. Life was so hectic, I didn't even find time to buy a hat, so I bought a matching rose and pinned it to the navy blue wisp of a hat I'd worn when I first met Her Royal Highness. And just in case she had chosen to wear green, I took another dress with me on 'The Day', all set to do a quick change act if need be. But I needn't have worried.

When the Duchess arrived, she was wearing a most beautifully cut coat and a matching hat in the identical shade of yellow as our 'One In a Million' badges. Instinctively, I knew that her choice was intentional and not mere chance. This was so typically thoughtful of this gracious lady, whose warmth and sincerity I value so much.

I'm afraid I threw Pauline into a panic by asking her to use my ciné-camera to record the proceedings.

'Oh, my goodness, what if I make a mess of it?'

'You won't. You've handled it before. In any case, whatever you manage to film, it will be more than I can do. I can't be behind a ciné camera on this occasion, can I?'

As it turned out, we now have a filmed record of that happy day which has since given pleasure to so many people in the North West. People who had contributed to the Fund could now see the scanner they had helped to provide and, in some measure, share that memorable day. I later had it copied on video, for once the film was worn, it could not be replaced.

Escorted by Sir William Downward, Lord Lieutenant of Greater Manchester who is also the chairman of my Central Committee and one of the Trustees of my Fund and also by Mr Robert Prain, Chairman of the Manchester South (Teaching) Area Health Authority, the Duchess first met officials of the hospital on the forecourt and in the reception area, then met members of the nursing staff.

She then came to the new department, where the Director of Radiotherapy, Dr Robert Gibb, introduced Her Royal Highness to Doctors Ian Todd, David Greene and Brian Eddleston, all of whom are the technical members of my Central Committee. Dr Todd, Assistant Director of Radiotherapy hails from Scotland. Physicist Dr Greene is Irish and Dr Eddleston, Director of Diagnostic Radiology is a Lancastrian. During the ups and downs of the 'scanner trail' we had established a friendly rapport which included the occasional teasing and banter. I remember a conver-

54

sation with them just a couple of weeks before the big day about which we were all getting excited. They'd been teasing me about something – I forgot what – and my parting shot had been: 'Of course, you know how I intend to begin my speech, don't you?'

'No. How?'

'There was an Englishman, an Irishman and a Scotsman . . .' and walked out with a polite 'good afternoon, gentlemen' amid peals of laughter.

Next in the receiving line was Dr Godfrey Hounsfield, the inventor of the scanner and Nobel Prize winner who was later to be knighted by the Queen. I was so thrilled that he had found the time to share the day with us, for he had been with us when the foundation stone was laid and indeed he had helped to lay it. I was standing next in line and the Duchess greeted me with a kiss. I told her how very welcome she was. After being shown round the department and having had the complicated machinery, computers, consoles etc. explained to her by Dr Eddleston, the Duchess then signed the hospital's visitors' book, the Scanner Department's visitors' book and a copy of her official photograph. We then proceeded into the refectory, now bedecked with superb floral arrangements for the unveiling of the commemorative plaque, which was later to be fixed to the wall of the reception area of the department, together with the signed photograph.

As her father, Patrick Hayward, and her brother Peter looked on, young Sacha Hayward stepped forward to present Her Royal Highness with a bouquet. Having been one of the first people to read One Day At a Time, the Duchess was well aware that Patrick and his late wife Julé had initiated our 'one in a million' badges, which has advanced the Fund by no less than a quarter of a million pounds. Oh, if only Julé could have shared the day with us. Bless her, she had only time to study the plans before she died of cancer. She didn't live to see one brick put on top of another, which to me is a great sorrow, considering the wonderful contribution she

55

made. I asked the Duchess if she would accept one of Julé's badges. She took it from my hand, and, giving it to Sacha, asked her to pin it on her coat. To watch that little girl pin her Mummy's badge on the Duchess's coat was a most poignant moment. It was as much as I could do to prevent myself bursting into tears.

Then came the speeches.

Amid camera flashlight bulbs, whirring TV cameras and a forest of microphones, Mr Prain welcomed Her Royal Highness and invited her to unveil the plaque. Having done so, she then spoke to the assembled company. The Duchess, referring to me, said:

'She is a crusader of courage and by her indomitable spirit and her belief in the good of human nature – which I share with her – none of us have been able to resist the call of this Pied Piper.' She concluded with the words: 'I am the lucky one today, for saying publicly the words so many people would like to say personally: "Pat Seed, thank you."'

I then told those present of the Duchess's personal involvement with, and contribution to the Fund and said that there was no person I would rather have to open it than HRH The Duchess of Kent. Equally as important as the fact that the Christie had a scanner was the spirit which had made it possible. It was the same spirit which had taken on the Spanish Armada and, in the dark days of the last war, had taken on the might of the German Luftwaffe to win the Battle of Britain. It was the community spirit I remembered as a child during the Manchester and Salford blitz. It was a spirit which ignored or bypassed all barriers – age, sex, race, creed, colour and political affiliations. My personal reward was the affection, comradeship and friendship which had come my way because of the Appeal. For me, it was a day of thanksgiving.

The formalities concluded, the Duchess then met and talked with as many people as time would allow. My dear old friend Minnie Hall was there in her wheelchair, accompanied by a member of the Salvation Army.

The Duchess held the hand of this indomitable old lady for a long time and promised: 'I'll come to see you when you are a hundred.' The look of astonishment and pure joy on Minnie's face was indescribable. She also had a special word for Stephen Bilynskyj, my young friend from Oldham. Stephen, who was blinded as the result of a mugging incident in his teens, had raised £700 by doing a sponsored swim for the Fund. A favourite with us all, no fund affair was complete without him. Later, as we were having lunch, I asked Her Royal Highness if she would please consider being a Patron, not of my Fund, but of the Hospital. To this she very graciously consented, but of course, it did have to go through official channels and it was some months later when Mr Prain was able to announce publicly that the Duchess of Kent is Patron of the Christie Hospital and Holt Radium Institute. It has given much pleasure to the entire hospital staff, the patients and to all the many people connected with the hospital.

As Her Royal Highness was leaving, to fulfil another engagement in Manchester, the patients and many members of staff lined the corridors, the reception area and the forecourt. Her visit had given so much pleasure to so many people, not least, to me. It left an aura of goodwill and what I can only describe as a feeling of 'togetherness' which lingered for many weeks to come.

Since that memorable day, our Royal Patron has paid a private visit to the hospital, to see in greater detail the many facets of the work. I know that she would never be content to be Patron in name only, for it is not in her nature to do so. Hers is a sincere and total commitment and the Christie has, in the Duchess of Kent, a lifelong friend.

6

THE MONTH OF May came and went, during which I visited many parts of the North West. Then, in the first week of June, I went to Berkshire, thus keeping my promise to Ken Thomas and staying for a week with relatives of mine who were then living in Maidenhead.

Until then, Ken had been a 'telephone friend' and it was a pleasure to meet this burly, affable man and his charming wife Polly and also members of various Berkshire fund raising groups. Ken's personal charisma, his boundless enthusiasm and dedication were infectious. He was bubbling over with plans and ideas and so far had managed to beat his six month deadline. To look at him in those days of summer, nobody would have guessed that he was living under a death sentence – unless you knew how much his efforts and his public appearances took out of him. I did. For every hour he spent in the public eye, an hour was spent flat on his back, trying to recoup and harness his waning strength. He had arranged a full programme of events for me to attend and on two occasions I was able to show my ciné film of the C.A.T. scanner at the Christie. Until you have actually seen just what this incredible technology will do, the word 'scanner' – although you know it is something worthwhile – does not mean very much to you. Now, many of the Berkshire fund raisers could see for themselves the target to which their efforts were directed. However, I must admit, it tickled my sense of humour to find that Reading is the constituency of the Minister of Health, Dr Gerard Vaughan. It was a happy and pleasant week in which I made many new friends and at the end of it came home sure in the knowledge that their appeal would some day reach a successful conclusion. I have two treasured souvenirs of that happy week – a cut glass tumbler on which are engraved the crow and the thorn, thus denoting 'Crowthorne' and a huge greetings card signed by all the children from various Berkshire schools who attended a Children's Rally. Ken's devotion to children equalled my own and he found as I had found, that children were among his most enthusiastic supporters. Adverse comments by Job's comforters in the local press worried him, but I told him to ignore them and get on with the job. Happily, they were very much a minority, for most of the Berkshire Press gave him excellent support.

Back home again, two events stand out in my mind before my family and I made our annual visit to Trearddur Bay. The first was an invitation to the school I'd attended as a junior, Halton Bank School. Anyone who has read *One Day At a Time* will know that I was the headmistress's *bête noire*, I felt sure that if she were able to see *me* opening the summer fair, it would be enough to make her turn in her grave. However, my lifelong friend Beryl Acton rang round several of our former classmates and it became something of an old girls' reunion. As we toured the various classrooms (how *small* they seemed) it began a string of 'D'you remember the day when. . . .' A nostalgic trip forty years down memory lane. Headmaster Mr Alan Robinson was a courteous host and later I received a very handsome cheque from the school and the P.T.A.

The second engagement which stands out in my mind also concerns a school – St Michael's High School, Chorley, where one of the first-year tutorials is named after me. I was invited to present the prizes at Speech Day on 4th July.

Parents, pupils and staff were gathered in the hall and a side table groaned under the weight of trophies and prizes for various academic and sporting achievements. As boys and girls came to the dais to receive their awards, the array on the side table dwindled. Then, headmaster Mr Moore explained to those assembled that I had given a silver tray, suitably inscribed, as a trophy for the boy or girl who had contributed most to the quality of the life of the school or the local community. Whilst he was doing so, the master in charge of the trophies was saying to me, sotto voce: 'I can't find it. What does it look like?'

I explained. I couldn't see it, either.

Mr Moore then turned to me with a smile, obviously expecting me to hand over the tray to the two girls who were to share the award.

'I'm so glad to have the winners here tonight. Unfortunately, we can't find the tray,' I said, goodhumouredly.

And nor did we. Mr Moore was most concerned and vanished from the hall at a rate of knots to look for it. None of the staff left that night until the tray was eventually found beneath a pile of papers. It had been taken from its 'safe place' for cleaning and had been inadvertently hidden.

The headmaster was most concerned in case I should be upset or offended, but I could only see the funny side of it.

'Don't worry about it,' I told him, 'There's one thing, those children aren't likely to forget the year I gave the prizes, are they?' I know that if I had been a child at that Speech Day, the missing prize would have made my night. Finally, Mr Moore had to admit that the incident did have its funny side. Ruefully I thought: 'It could only happen to me. If anything can go wrong – it will!'

As usual, I took my art materials to Trearddur and when the rest of the family were going for long walks, scrambling about the rocks, etc., I spent my time drawing and painting. It's a hobby for which I have very little time when at home. Then I had a bright idea. I designed six Christmas cards and on our return from holiday, had them printed. Later in the year the sale of them brought in about £800 for the Fund.

August 9th 1980 . . . and another memorable day. Patrick Hayward's partner had enlisted the aid of his son, Simon Morton, in the distribution of our 'One In a Million' badges. One late afternoon, Simon was delivering badges to the home of Peter and Lillian Scott who run the Darwen branch of the Appeal. Lovable and motherly Lillian had invited Simon to stay for tea. That is how he came to meet their daughter, Karen, who, after the meal, helped Simon to deliver the rest of his consignment. It was the beginning of a romance for these two young people and I was delighted to think that the Appeal had inadvertently played Cupid. Therefore, when Geoff and I received an invitation to their wedding, we were more than happy to accept.

Lillian is a member of a large family and has seven children of her own. She also has a heart of gold. Of Scottish origin, many of the 'clan' turned up, including Uncle Tom – complete with kilt and sporran etc., – who was the life and soul of the party. After the speeches at the reception, plus some hilarious antics from Uncle Tom, who suddenly appeared with claymore and shield, looking as though he was all set to re-enact the massacre of Glencoe, the brides-maids presented their posies to the grandmothers.

'What a delightful gesture,' I thought – and then was quite overwhelmed when the bride came to present her bouquet to me.

'We wouldn't have met, but for you and the Appeal,' she whispered.

I was deeply moved. In the days which followed I sprayed Karen's bouquet with water to keep it fresh as long as possible. Before the flowers faded, I pressed one as a permanent souvenir. I have it still.

Talking of flowers, another nice compliment was to have a flower named after me. Grown by Mr Ron Nelson of Carnforth, it is a magnificent yellow dahlia, a vigorous healthy specimen which is reminiscent of our badges, and which measures some seven or eight inches across. It so

61

happened that one local newspaper reported the fact with a headline 'floral tribute to Pat Seed' which caused some of the community to think I'd departed this life!

On a sunny Saturday afternoon in September I went to an event in the Fylde village of Pilling. Organised mainly by Mrs Elsie Lawrenson, the entire village rallied and their combined efforts raised over £2,000 – in one afternoon. How they did it, I don't know, but they did. You would think that by now I would be used to such efforts, but the sheer undiluted goodwill of people and the results they produce, never ceases to amaze me.

It was the same at Congleton on 7th October. I had travelled some sixty miles down the M6 motorway in foul weather, to attend a function at the Prince of Wales Hotel. With a westerly gale behind driving rain, spray from the northbound carriageway was deluging the south bound lane and driving conditions were appalling. The warmth of the welcome from Mr Peter Edwards and his wife Phyllis and their clientele more than compensated. By events of various kinds, they had raised the grand sum of over £1,200. It was a festive night of good humour and generosity and on my return journey, I brought home a large iced cake (too big for the family, so given to our local old people's home) some flowers and a copper engraving of Congleton Town Hall. People like this really do make one wonder why there is so much strife in this world.

The 20th October – our 29th wedding anniversary – we spent in London. I had again been invited to the Women of the Year Luncheon at the Savoy and it was during the pre-lunch reception that the Marchioness of Lothian asked me if I would accept an 'honour' and said that she would be in touch with me.

That evening, my cousin Ann (who was my bridesmaid and is the nearest I have to a sister) and her husband David came with Geoff and me to the London Palladium. Topping the bill was my friend Ken Dodd. Backstage, later he offered us a celebratory drink. I had watched Ken at work many times. Northern audiences are readily appreciative of his quick wit. To watch him on one of the world's most famous stages cajole and captivate a cosmopolitan audience left me full of admiration for his professionalism. That audience were going to have their chuckle muscles titilated whether they liked it or not. And by golly, they did. Mind you, we four Lancastrians thought they were a bit slow on the uptake to start with. But, given a live audience, there are few that Ken cannot win over; for the umpteenth time in his career he had the London Palladium eating out of his hand.

Back home again and just seven days later, life was no laughing matter for many Lancashire people. Some of the highest tides of the year coincided with incessant rain, draining tons of water off the hills to meet inflowing sea water. Something had to give – and did. The Fylde (the old English word for 'field') is a natural flood plain and the man made embankments of the River Wyre took intolerable pressure. In several places banks were breached and particularly hard hit was the tiny village of St Michaels. Thousands of acres of the North West were under several feet of water, bringing misery to countless families.

As I mentioned in *One Day At a Time* my husband is the North West Water Authority's Area Engineer (Rivers Division) for Central Lancashire. Geoff is a very caring person. Not only did he and his men witness several years work washed away, his heart went out to the victims of this natural disaster. Television, radio, the national and local Press reported the sequence of events and at St Michaels, the Army were called in to help. Adversity generally brings out the best in most people and co-operation became the order of the day, with good neighbourliness and good humour triumphing in spite of it all.

In nearly thirty years of marriage, I had witnessed similar situations, but none on quite this scale. My role at times like this is to man our emergency telephone, fill thermos flasks, make endless sandwiches for men who are working around the clock and to try to provide an instant hot meal for a

63

husband who may come in ten hours late to eat it. He comes home to snatch as little sleep as will enable him to continue the job. A couple of hours at the most, and he's off again. Three members of his family had their homes flooded at St Michaels.

I was left coping with the water flowing through our garage, trying to unblock drains choked with fallen autumn leaves, so that they might take the water which covered the garden like a lake. My son and I worked frantically to stop water, already at doorstep level, from coming into our home and it was touch and go whether we began taking up the carpets. Eventually, the turbulent elements quietened, flood water gradually subsided and weary farmers and householders began to count the cost. It had left in its wake a devastation amounting to millions of pounds' worth of damage, heartbreak for many and, for my husband and his colleagues, the mammoth task of repair and renewal. Little more than a year later, vast areas of Yorkshire were to suffer a similar fate.

In May I had received a letter from Professor Philip Reynolds, Vice Chancellor of the University of Lancaster, informing me that the Senate wished to confer upon me the Honorary Degree of M.A. I would be informed of the date in December when confirmation had been received from the Chancellor, the Princess Alexandra.

Later, I was notified that the congregation for the conferment of Higher and Honorary Degrees would take place on the 2nd. On the evening 1st December, Geoff and I were invited to dinner at the University, given by the Senate in honour of the honorands. They included historian Sir Roger Fulford and Mr Bill Opher CBE, the joint Managing Director of Vickers Ltd of Barrow-in-Furness. It was a thoroughly enjoyable and pleasant evening; excellent food, stimulating conversation and interesting speeches. This time, I could just sit back, relax and enjoy it all, knowing that not too much was demanded of me, for Mr Opher replied on behalf of the honorands. As one who has had a long and

64

close association with the University of Lancaster, he knew most of those present extremely well, so that his scintillating wit included some 'in' jokes which received a very appreciative reception. During dinner, I asked the Vice Chancellor, somewhat diffidently, what one was supposed to do with an Honorary MA, adding that I didn't consider myself to be an academic.

'There are forms of achievement other than those of an academic nature,' replied Professor Reynolds, 'After tomorrow's ceremony you will be an MA of this University. We will be most offended if you do not use it. We will expect you to put the letters M.A. after your name.'

'Not *HON* MA?'

'No. Just M.A.'

The next day, Geoff and I were at the University for lunch with Princess Alexandra and her Lady in Waiting the Lady Mary Fitzalan Howard.

I was delighted to meet them again. The last time I had been in their company was when Her Royal Highness had come especially to Lancaster Town Hall and had done me the honour of presenting me with the Lancaster 'Citizen of the Year' Award, which is promoted by the *Lancaster Guardian*. During lunch I also met Mr Colin Lyas, the lecturer who was to give the oration in support of me.

After lunch, suitably robed, we all proceeded into the great hall of the University, to a fanfare of trumpets by the trumpeters of Lancashire Constabulary. When we were all seated on the platform, I am told that it was a most impressive sight. In the centre Her Royal Highness was seated, wearing the magnificent red and gold robe of Chancellor and a black velvet plumed hat. On her right were the three Pro-Chancellors: Lord Taylor of Blackburn, Sir Alastair Pilkington and Mr Cyril Smith, MP. I was seated next to this ample Member of Parliament and I have to confess that I dared not move, for Cyril occupied not only his own chair, but half of mine. On the other side of me was Sir Roger, well over eighty years of age and somewhat infirm. I was terrified of sending him crashing to the floor.

The body of the hall was occupied by those who were to receive higher degrees and these were bestowed first. Then came the honorary degrees. Each of us in turn had to stand whilst the orator presented us to Her Royal Highness. Mr Lyas, who lectures in Philosophy, gave my biographical details and spoke of the progress of the Appeal Fund, ending with the words 'Honoris causa'. I walked the few paces to stand before the Chancellor to whom I made a formal bow, after which she presented me with the red cylindrical leather case which contained my degree. It was embossed in gold lettering: The University of Lancaster.

Amid applause, the Princess asked me:

'Where is your husband?'

'Sitting in the gallery, Ma'am.'

For Geoff it was an occasion which filled him with pride and my little Mother, who had been so thrilled by the entire proceedings, was moved to tears. As for me, a woman whose secondary education had been impaired by wartime circumstances, it was one of the proudest moments of my life. How I envy today's students their opportunities to study whatever subjects interest them. Were I not so committed, I would dearly like to read English language and Literature and possibly study the origin of language. Maybe . . . one day.

On the way home, Geoff said that he was beginning to wonder to whom he was married.

'Don't you *dare* think like that. Anyway, right now, my love, I'm thinking about what I'm going to give you for dinner!'

However, I knew what he meant, for I couldn't help thinking, 'Is this really happening to me?'

Meanwhile, I had heard from Lady Lothian, herself a distinguished journalist, that the honour to which she had referred at the Women of the Year Luncheon was no less than the Valiant For Truth Media Award – the highest award any journalist can hope to receive. Known to all her

66

friends as Tony, Antonella, Marchioness of Lothian is the Chairman of the Advisory Council which includes the names of some of the most eminent 'top brass' in television, radio and the newspaper industry. I had been voted the 1980 recipient.

Given by The Order of Christian Unity of which Lady Lothian is the president, previous winners of the Award include distinguished people such as Oliver Whiteley, architect of the BBC World Service; Baroness Jackson of Lodsworth; Ross McWhirter (posthumously); Anatol Goldberg; Dr Sheila Cassidy and Dr Conor Cruise O'Brien. Each year the presentation has been made at the International Press Club, London and equally notable people have made the presentation – ballerina Beryl Grey OBE; Group Captain Leonard Cheshire, VC; Sir Charles Curran; Jane Ewart Biggs and Lord Barnetson. The Award consists of a simple wooden shield on which is inscribed a quotation from John Bunyan's *Pilgrim's Progress*. It is a 'no money' award. To quote Lady Lothian:

'Many ask why it was founded by an interdenominational association of Christians. First, as Bunyan so usefully reminds us, courage and accuracy are not only essential human ethics, they are also essential Christian ethics. We believed that it was time that outstanding achievements by media men and women should be recognised. At the same time, because Truth and Courage do have many faces, year by year we have seen both these ethics most clearly conveyed when strikingly contrasted to the recurring background of falsehood and fear. These two trials, all winners of the Award have overcome.'

On 15th December 1980 my family and my close personal friends went to the London Press Club. Amid TV lights and cameras, microphones and tape recorders, it was the proudest moment of my life when Sheila Scott OBE, the first woman to fly solo over the North Pole (in addition to three times solo round the world) and the holder of a hundred flying records, presented me with my shield. The citation reads: 'For shining like a lamp of courage for all who fear cancer and using her skill as a journalist to communicate how she overcame pain and illness *One Day At a Time* – the title of her autobiography.'

My beloved friend, the Right Reverend Anthony Hoskyns-Abrahall, the former Anglican Bishop of Lancaster, concluded the presentation with a reflection.

'As St Paul said, spiritual things are spiritually discerned. Miracles demand a costly co-operation of faith, truth and surrender. Pat came to her anointing (The Sacrament of the Anointing of the Sick) not as a spiritual refugee looking for a handout, but as a soldier of Christ to be briefed for the battle which lay ahead.'

Later in his speech, the Bishop used favourite words of mine, from the writings of St Theresa of Avila:

Christ has
No body now on earth but yours;
No hands but yours;
No feet but yours.
Yours are the eyes
Through which is to look out
Christ's compassion to the World;
Yours are the feet with which He is to go about
Doing good;
Yours are the hands
With which He is to bless men now.

I do not intend to give here a resumé of all the speeches, for they are set out in booklet form and available from The Order of Christian Unity. It was a great personal pleasure to have so many members of the media present to share the occasion with me, for many of them had given me invaluable help.

To mention them all is impossible, but they included my friend Jean Rook; Stan Blenkinsop, Northern news editor of the *Daily Express*; Duncan Measor, diarist of the *Man-*

chester Evening News; Brian Hargreaves, editor of the *West Lancashire Evening Gazette*; Ben Fisher, the *Lancashire Evening Post*'s 'John Preston'; Tom Scott, former editor of the *Lancaster Guardian* and many more. Personal guests, included my district nurse and friend Marie Calvert and her husband Eddie; two of our Garstang clergy, the Reverend Eric Carter, vicar of our parish church and the Reverend Father Conway, priest of St Mary & Michaels RC church; my good friends Bobby and Norma Charlton. Also there were Rona Randall and her husband Freddie; Kay Fisher and her daughters Susan (our god-daughter) and Hazel; Geoffrey Ball, the treasurer of my Fund and, from the Christie, Dr and Mrs David Greene. My son Michael recorded the occasion with his camera. Last, but not least, the man who has sustained me with his unfailing love and support, my beloved husband Geoffrey.

Later that evening, the 'Garstang Gang' headed north again, courtesy of British Rail. It had been a long day, but the journeys to and from London had been enlivened with laughter and repartee.

In the cloakroom at the Press Club a charming gentleman had helped my incorrigible Marie to take off her velvet jacket.

'Now mind what you're doing with that. It's a bit of good stuff. We're not all scruffs in Lancashire, you know!' The gentleman smilingly assured her that he would personally guarantee that her jacket would come to no harm. As he walked away, Marie asked: 'Who was that?'

I assumed a pained expression and looked at the ceiling in mock exasperation. '*Only* Lord Lothian. Honestly, I can take you anywhere twice – the second time to apologise!'

But Marie's personality is such that she can get away with murder (although that's hardly the right term to use about a district nurse). On the homeward journey she came in for plenty of teasing and Father Conway said that he had long since given up with her. (I knew that priest and nurse had a high regard for each other.) Completely undaunted, she

69

told us that she had turned up half an hour late for her wedding, but Father Conway still had her and Eddie out of church on time. It was all good fun, with the two clergymen exchanging banter which kept us all laughing. There's nothing wrong with our Christian Unity in Garstang and a very happy day it had been.

I have appreciated and I value all the many honours which have been bestowed upon me.

Yet, Valiant For Truth is so very special. It's the only honour I have ever displayed on the wall of my sitting room. I know that other recipients feel as I do, that this is an Award which one can have on view without feeling 'big headed'.

Why?

Several reasons. First, because of the symbol of the Order of Christian Unity – hands joined in friendship at the foot of the Cross. Those of the Order, of which I am now a member, put Jesus Christ and His teaching before all else. The fact that they may be Church of England, Roman Catholic, Methodist Church of Scotland or of the Salvation Army is secondary. Although there is a respect for each denomination's interpretation and application of the Christian Faith, the emphasis is on the things which unite us rather than aspects which divide us. There is also a positive approach to the 20th century problems about which we can work *together*.

Secondly, I know that the members of the Advisory Council who nominated me for the Award may appreciate more than most people my parallel battle against ill health and my relentless pursuit of my objective. For example, Lady Lothian who is one of the most totally committed Christians I know, lost an eye through cancer. Vivienne Plummer of Granada Television, also a member of the Council, said to me: 'I might not have a husband, but for the scanner.' At Granada TV in Manchester, Peter Plummer, a Christie patient, is now back at work as a programme producer.

And when I look at the quotation inscribed on my shield,

70

I am comforted, for it conveys no more and no less than the Truth:

I do not repent me of all the trouble I
have been at, to arrive where I am.

John Bunyan.

7

1980 DREW TO A close. Between Christmas and New Year I had a depressing feeling of unease. I had got through almost four years . . . would I reach that 'five years cancer free' milestone? Or would something go wrong on the last lap?

Dear Marie, who at a professional level is unequalled, watches over me like a hen with one chick.

'I'm always glad when you've got New Year's Eve over, then I feel you can relax,' she says, remembering that other New Year's Eve when I was on the operating table at the Christie. Yet the feeling of foreboding persisted and it must have been some kind of premonition, for the first part of 1981 was the saddest period of the Appeal.

It began with a call from Pauline Worthington who, with her mother Mrs Barnett, runs the Stockport branch of the Fund. She told me that my old friend Minnie Hall had died and that the funeral was on 2nd January. Dear Minnie had, as her fellow Salvationists put it, been called to higher service. Indeed, her funeral service was a celebration of that fact. I remembered her, physically frail and wheelchair bound at the opening of the CAT Department. Since the Duchess of Kent had promised to visit her when she was one hundred, this, Pauline Worthington told me, had grown in Minnie's mind to a full scale party for her at Buckingham

Palace. But it wasn't to be. In her youth she had been one of the famous Tiller Girls but had given up the glitter of the stage in order, to use her own words, 'to sing for God'. From the window of her ground floor flat she had persuaded passers-by to put something in her 'Pat Seed tin'. By this means, this indominable old lady had raised almost £1,000. After the Duchess had shaken her hand, anyone else who wanted that privilege had to pay 10p – into her tin! I felt her loss deeply. She was 88 years of age. A good innings but isn't it always too soon to lose someone you love?

Then came a call from Berkshire. Ken Thomas, who had spent the last year of his life on his own 'scanner trail' had died on New Year's Day, having raised almost half a million pounds. I could not attend his funeral, but in late February, Pauline and I travelled to Reading and at St Mary's Parish Church his memorial service was conducted by his friend and counsellor, the Reverend C. Hadley. I was privileged to offer a reading from *Pilgrim's Progress*. In his final letter to me, Ken had written to say that both his sons were engaged to be married, which was a great joy to him. He also said that he was thinking of getting some kind of caravan so that he could travel lying down to ease the pain. For sheer guts, I have met few men to equal him and I will always be proud to have known him.

Back home, I had a call from Darwen to tell me that Peter, Lillian Scott's husband, had died of a massive heart attack. Thinking back to the day of Karen and Simon's wedding and of the happiness of this large united family, it seemed unbelievable. Peter had been a cancer patient and like me, had been 'doing nicely' until his untimely demise from a quite different and unexpected cause. How I grieved for them. And for myself, too. I had lost three good friends and I loved them all.

1981 and The International Year of the Disabled. I was reminded of a hymn I'd written some years ago, to which my friend Allan Burnham-Airey had written a melody.

73

All men everywhere need a hand
At some time or another.
Do we care? Do you care
For fellow man, your brother?
Safely in our own small world,
Is it enough to say
Your problem's no concern of mine
Please be on your way.

The simpler choice to turn aside,
Leave someone else to cope.
But if we stop to offer help
Then for us all there's hope.
So will you give that helping hand?
Your brother's in distress.
It's not enough to stand and say:
'This world is in a mess'.

Sharing more and caring more,
That's what we all must do.
Be tireless and unsparing, too,
To help each other through.
To love our neighbour as ourselves
As children we were told.
And if we do – yes, me and you,
Peace will then unfold.

So many disabled people had contributed to my Fund that I
felt I must help in some way. In my youth, I had aspirations
to be a channel swimmer, but in those days the reception
committee at Cap Gris Nez would have been a contingent of
the German Army.

However, swimming was something I could still do, so I
offered to do a sponsored swim in aid of the Lord Mayor of
Manchester's project for International Year of the Disabled.
On 26th of February, I went to Sharston Baths, Wythen-
shawe where I was joined by Mandy Kyffin and Michael
Kenny, both of them Paraplegic Olympic Gold Medalists.

74

The objective was a mere 100 metres – enough for me at 52. I am not ashamed to say that both Mandy and Mike left me floundering. I came in last! Not that it was a race. It was a joy to see the freedom of movement these two young people gained in the water. And as I swam, I thought fondly of Stephen, my blind young friend from Oldham who had raised £700 with his sponsored swim.

I could not have known that it was at almost exactly that moment when his mother, Mary Bilynskyj found him dead in bed. Tall, handsome and with an albino fairness, Stephen had heart trouble. Now, it had just stopped beating. It would be about 5 p.m. when the phone rang. It was my friend Barbara Dignan, chairman of the Oldham branch of the Fund.

'Pat, are you by yourself or is someone with you?'

'My son is at home, Barbara. Why?'

'Sit down. I've got some awful news . . .'

Blind though he was, this courageous young man had picked up the threads of life and made the best of it. Like any other lad of his age, he wanted to be independent and he had a flat of his own. Across the road and from the windows of their flat, his parents could keep an eye on him. When it had got to past eleven o'clock that morning and Mary had not seen Stephen knocking about in his kitchen, she had gone to see if he was all right. Only to find him dead. He was just twenty-three.

At his funeral the church was packed. Bobby Charlton, who had taken a personal interest in Stephen, taking him to Manchester United's Club at Old Trafford, attended the service. How we grieved for the loss of his young life and how all of us connected with the Fund would miss him. He had been a favourite of us all and we had included him in everything we did.

On 28th May I was invited to attend a service in Westminster Abbey to mark the Diamond Jubilee of the Greater London Fund for the Blind.

Mary Bilynskyj accompanied me. The service of re-

75

dedication and thanksgiving had for us the dual purpose of being a memorial service for Stephen. We were seated in the South Lantern. Just in front of the sanctuary and beyond the choristers' stalls, HRH The Duchess of Kent was seated.

It was a most moving service and as the organ and voices soared, Mary, who had not been in Westminster Abbey before, said to me:

'It's like being in heaven, isn't it? I do wish Stephen were here to see this.'

'What makes you think he can't, Mary. I'm sure he will know. And I'm sure he would not want you to grieve any more. Be happy, for his sake. It is what he would want.'

I prayed that the all pervading peace of this historic holy place would enter the soul of Mary and help her to come to terms with her loss.

I think it would be March when Bert Brierley first told me that he had leukemia. Big, ebullient extrovert generous Bert, the man who had started my 'scanner trail' off with the first £1000. The man who was convinced that providing a scanner could be done, when most people thought I was crackers.

'I know you'll do it. You'll confound the sceptics. I recognise determination when I see it. You and I came out of a similar mould.'

How Bert – and Stephen – had enjoyed themselves at 'This Is Your Life'. How proud they had been to meet the Duchess of Kent at the Royal opening of that scanner department.

One of Bert's several companies was a garden centre, 'Garstang Gardens'. In the small garden outside the scanner building, my magnolia tree flourished. It was a present from the Manchester Junior Chamber of Commerce and Trade when I was Mancunian of the Year. I rang Bert to ask if he could find me some yellow roses for my garden.

'Yes, and I know just which variety. I'll bring you a dozen

'Belle Blonde' in tribute to that bonny Royal lass who opened the building for you.'

That had been in the autumn of 1980.

Now Bert, like his late wife Phyllis, had a form of cancer.

Bert and I were of the same comparatively rare blood group – AB positive, yet ironically, I couldn't help him, for cancer patients are not allowed to donate blood.

There are many types of leukemia, some curable, some controllable, some of slow progression and others virulent and rapidly progressive. Marie and I visited Bert in his room at the Christie to find him with sketch pad and pencil, re-designing his plastic isolation tent. It was typical of this imaginative, inventive man.

'This damn thing is no bloody good!' he said and proceeded to tell us what was wrong with it and how it could be improved.

'Some of the doctors are in America, looking at the latest isolation tents. They're about £5,000 a throw. If they think they are any good, I'll start them off with half a dozen.'

And he would have done, had he lived. In spite of every effort, modern medicine had no answer with which to halt the rapid destruction of Bert's blood cells. On 1st May, he died. Garstang had lost one of its 'characters' and I had lost a loyal friend.

What a year it had been. I had reached the stage of wondering which of my friends I would lose next. I seemed to be in a permanent state of apprehension and I wasn't sleeping very well. Then, like a ray of sunshine, came a bright note which raised my spirits.

Attending a function in Chorley, one of the ladies said to me:

'D'you remember little Claire, the two-year-old who presented you with a bouquet when you attended the Tug of War?'

Oh yes, I remembered the little mite in the pretty smocked dress and the lace mob cap which hid the fact that she hadn't any hair, due to her treatment for cancer of the kidney. My heart sank . . . *oh no, not Claire as well* . . . 'I'm sure you'll be glad to know that she's doing fine. The doctors say that it isn't likely that there will be a recurrence of her trouble. She's five years old now and at school.'

'I'm so delighted to hear that. I seem to have lost so many good friends this year. Do you see her family? Would you ask her Mummy if I could please have a picture of Claire?'

A week or so later, Mrs Ainscough *and* Claire wrote to me, enclosing a picture of the prettiest little poppet with shoulder length blonde shining hair and a shy smile. In her hands she clasped what I should think is her favourite dolly.

'I'm having that framed,' I told Pauline. 'It's going on the desk, and whenever things go wrong or we are tempted to say "sod it!", we'll look at little Claire and know that what we are doing is worthwhile. She can be our mascot.'

I look at her picture as I write. I cannot help but smile back at her.

Can you imagine standing on a pavement in Stoke-on-Trent at 4 o'clock in the morning; beside you is a great big drum. As you stand there in your evening dress, shivering in the early morning air, round the corner come two policemen and a policewoman, who eye you with appraising looks, tinged with suspicion. No? Well, it happened to me.

I greeted the triple arm of the law with:

'It's not mine. It's Ken Dodd's,' indicating the drum.

It all started when I got to know Mrs Phyllis Ford. Phyllis had a dress business in Stoke-on-Trent and it was when she came to Manchester, buying, that she saw one of the Fund's collecting boxes in one of the dress warehouses. She asked what it was – and went home and started an Appeal for a scanner for the Stoke-on-Trent area. After an exchange of letters and several phone conversations we had met in Manchester one morning in February. A couple of weeks later, Phyllis and her husband Frank had come to the Christie to see the scanner department. A generous hearted and caring couple, Phyllis and Frank have a lively sense of humour. Later, at their invitation, I visited the Royal Doulton Beswick factory with them and with Ken Dodd, who is also Patron of the Stoke Appeal. On the occasion when I was standing on the pavement with Ken's drum it was the end of a fund-raising evening at Jollee's Night Club when Ken had topped the bill. He hadn't come off stage until 2 a.m. and by the time all the people who wanted to meet him had left his dressing room and all his props were stowed in his car, it was past four in the morning when we all went back to Frank and Phyllis's home for a meal. We sat talking until 5.30 a.m. That's when Ken decided it was time to make tracks for Knotty Ash. He had to be at Burtonwood the next day at lunch time. I just do not know where that man finds all his energy. As for me, I crawled into my sleeping bag on one of Phyllis's spare beds and knew nothing until midday.

Then I had contact with yet another 'scanner trailer'.

In Lanarkshire, Mrs Ilse Youngman had been treated for cancer. She was prepared to write a substantial cheque in appreciation of the excellent care she had received. But her doctors at Belvedere Hospital asked instead that she come back in twelve months when she had recovered and re-gained her strength, *then* they would tell her how she could help. This was how Ilse learned of the CT scanner and how it could benefit cancer patients.

Ilse read my book but for a long long time hesitated to contact me. The reason? She is German by birth and in my book is a graphic description of the German Blitzkrieg of Manchester. Eventually, she did telephone me, diffident and almost apologetic.

'Oh, Ilse, the war was forty years ago. We can't go on living in the past. That part of the book was intended to convey the community spirit which prevailed at that time. Anyway, the people of Essen and Dresden probably weren't too happy when the RAF bombed *them*.'

As with other 'scanner trailers' in various parts of Britain,

I found that Ilse and I were on the same wavelength. Later, she and a party of her committee members, including some of the medical staff of the hospital, drove from Lanarkshire to visit me. Ilse stayed with us and the rest of the party were accommodated locally. At my home, we talked until late evening. It proved to be an exchange of information, experience and ideas. I had the added bonus of having made another new friend. The next morning, we drove to Manchester, to the Christie Hospital, where they were able to see the scanner department in action. At this point, I left the Lanarkshire team in the capable hands of Dr Eddleston, for as always when I am at the hospital, I try to fit in as much as possible. I had a full day of appointments, including a meeting of the Central Committee and with my medical fitted in, somewhere along the line.

At Royal Doulton, I had been given a lovely model of a puma and I had bought a model of Red Rum for Bert Brierley as a reminder of the day he had taken me to meet the famous racehorse. I had intended to give it to him when he came out of hospital. But it wasn't to be. Now, I look at it with fond memories of a good and generous friend.

It was about this time that I paid a routine visit to my G.P. My dear doctor friend asked, conversationally:

'What are you and Geoff doing for a holiday this year?'

'Nothing much. We've got a rather special holiday planned for next February though.'

'*Next February*? That's nearly a year away. Now look here, Pat, Geoff has had a hell of a winter with all this flooding. As for you . . . well, you never did know how to pace yourself. Unless you come and tell me that you have booked a couple of weeks somewhere, I'm going to badger the pair of you until you do. Healthwise, it's a sound investment and I know that both of you are in need of a break.'

I came home, sat down and wondered where we could go. I knew he meant what he said. Anyway, you don't argue with an irate Scottish doctor, even if he is your friend. Then I had a bright idea. When Geoff came home I asked: 'How d'you fancy a trip to Vancouver?'

'*What*! Whose idea is this?'

'Don't blame me,' I grinned. 'It's doctor's orders.'

'Is it now? Did he say we could have it on the National Health?'

'Highly unlikely.'

My husband and Canadian Noel Beaumont had been the crew of a Mosquito aircraft in the Desert Air Force during the war. Since those days, when a friendship was formed which would last a lifetime, Noel and his wife Kay had visited us several times and we'd had repeated invitations to visit them in British Columbia.

'Let's go. If it's convenient for Noel and Kay to have us, then let's go. There are no pockets in a shroud. If this year has convinced me of anything, it is that we should do the things we want to do while we have the strength to do them. It's no good waiting until you are past it and then thinking of all the things that might have been. Anyway, who wants to be the richest corpse in the cemetery?' And in late August, we took flight – to beautiful British Columbia.

It was the break we needed. Neither of us realised just how much we needed it until we came home. It had taken a wise doctor to call the tune for us and we were glad and grateful that we had taken his advice.

8

EARLY IN 1981, the Order of Christian Unity had asked me to write a contribution to a book which they were to publish in the autumn. Its title was to be *Light in the Darkness – Disabled Lives*. I had written so much about cancer and as journalists will, I looked for a 'new angle'. 'Light' and 'dark' reminded me of the many people of other colours and cultures in Britain who had contributed to my Fund. It doesn't matter whether your skin is black, white or coffee coloured. If you have cancer, then you are all in the same predicament. And whatever the colour of your skin, every human being bleeds red blood. I know that my dear friend Bert Brierley wouldn't have cared two hoots if the donor came from Tottenham or Timbuctoo, if only his or her blood could have saved him. *Every* human being's basic need is to be loved; so, 'Love is a Many Splendoured Thing' became my contribution to 'Light in the Darkness'.

Then in July came the Toxteth riots. Like most people in Britain I felt very disturbed – and helpless.

When my daughter and her husband were at Liverpool University, they had a flat in Toxteth. I remembered that many Toxteth people had shown them small kindnesses and I knew that they were certainly not *all* rioters. I had bought the Victorian mahogany desk, at which I write, at the recently burnt out Rialto warehouse, which, in its heyday, had been a cinema.

I thought: 'Someone ought to do *something*!' – and then that inner voice replies: 'What about you? Why don't you think of something?' This, together with the thought that it is no use writing pieces such as 'Love is a Many Splendoured Thing' if, when put to the test, you haven't the guts to practise your convictions.

I telephoned several Liverpool councillors, including the then Lord Mayor whom I had met at a recent dinner at the Adelphi Hotel. He offered to help in any way he could. The general advice was 'keep out of it, the situation is too volatile.' Eventually I was given the name of the Warden of the Rialto Community Centre which is next to the burned shell of the former Rialto cinema. I telephoned him and arranged to go to see him.

I liked Ron Gilkes instantly. Here was a dedicated intelligent man, working as much as an eighty-hour week, in charge of a centre which included all age groups from a baby crêche to an OAP Club. People of this part of Liverpool's cosmopolitan population use it and as Ron put it;

'We take no account of people's colour, politics or religion. Everybody is welcome.'

'That's as it should be,' I replied and as we smiled at each other, his white teeth contrasted with his brown eyes and skin. Ron comes from Barbados. The last thing I wanted was to give the impression of being an interfering 'do gooder'. I genuinely wanted to help in a practical way. I told Ron of my special interest in children and he told me of his youth club.

Looking out of his office window at the piece of waste land on the other side of Upper Parliament Street, I asked:

'Ron, if we could get the use of that former bombed site over there, could you make use of it?'

'Sure we could. We have no outdoor facilities here, nowhere for the kids to play.'

The Centre is three old houses knocked into one – well-used, spotlessly clean and, a hive of activity.

'Right. Let's see how we get on. And if we do get it, let's

plant a garden and have a bit of colour to cheer up people.'

I came home and rang Liverpool's City Surveyor and told him what I had in mind.

He said that part of the site was scheduled for building, some time in the future but that he didn't see why it could not be used in the interim. I thanked him very much (before he could change his mind) and then rang the Parks Department to ask if they could possibly deliver a load of top soil. Having heard why it was required, they readily agreed. I telephoned Ron to tell him the news and we arranged a date when the children of the youth club would help the two of us to plant the garden.

Remembering the lovely story of the origin of the famous 'Peace' rose and knowing that nothing constructive or worthwhile is achieved in any sphere unless there is peace, I scrounged four Peace rose bushes and some bedding plants – red geraniums (Liverpool FC's colour) some blue lobelia (Everton FC) and also some yellow tagetes. I bought some gardening tools – a spade, a fork, a rake and a small trowel and fork, which came to just over £19. I admit that I did wonder if I was wasting my money, but the following morning a cheque came in for some writing I'd done and it was for . . . yes, just over £19. If the 'Scanner Trail' was full of coincidences, here was yet another. It convinced me that the thing was right.

A few days later, Tess Pickford and I loaded up the car and headed for Toxteth. The Parks Department brought not one, but four loads of top soil. In old slacks and wellies, I joined Ron and about twenty of his youngsters aged between seven and thirteen years of age. We raked and spaded the soil into a circular shape and in the centre, planted the Peace rose bushes and the geraniums. We then gave each boy or girl clumps of tagetes and lobelia – to make a yellow circle of colour and with the lobelia on the perimeter.

When the children were satisfied that the plants were evenly spaced, I had them gather round me, so that I could show them how to 'bed' their plants, telling them with a grin,

that you handle plants the same way you handle children –
gently, but firmly!

'Now, d'you think you could do that with your plants?'

When it was finished, they raked the soil smooth and Ron
found some bricks with which to border it and contain the
plot. As we stood back and surveyed our flower bed, a little
chap of seven or eight put his hand in mine.

'Are you pleased with your handiwork?'

'Yes, miss. Isn't it pretty?' he said, and then added, 'but
you know, somebody will have pinched them by tomorrow.'

Dear God, what an observation from one of such tender
years! All I could think of to say was:

'Have you enjoyed planting them today?'

'Ooh . . . yes!'

'Then nobody can take *that* away from you. If somebody
pinches them tomorrow, let's hope that they enjoy the
flowers, too.'

A few days later, I rang Ron. Yes, the garden was still
intact. A lot of passers-by had stopped to look at it. He said
he thought it was giving a lot of pleasure and he described it
as an oasis of colour in a brick desert.

Miraculously, nobody vandalised our little garden. It
flourished until the flowers faded in the autumn. Part of the
site was then taken over by builders who were to construct
flats for the Young People's Housing Association. They
kindly offered to bulldoze the remainder of the site for the
Community Centre. Say it with flowers? All Ron and I had
tried to do was to show that someone did care and that it is
more satisfying to build than to destroy.

In the summer of 1981 I received a letter from a consultant at the Christie who specialised in ear, nose and
throat disorders. He told me of a relatively new technology,
the CO_2 infra red laser for use in his particular branch of
surgery. Its advantages were indisputable and could the
Fund help?

This was discussed at our Central Committee meeting
and we agreed to provide the necessary finance – £25,000.

Maintenance and running costs over five years would amount to £4,500 which was about the amount raised by the New Speakers Club. The members are Christie patients who have had their voice box impaired or removed, which necessitates learning to speak from the diaphragm.

In late November, I was invited to see the laser in action. The specialist operated on a nine year old boy who had a crop of warts growing on his larynx, thus impairing his breathing and his voice. The child had gone through ten operations at his local general hospital.

In the operating theatre at the Christie he was prepared for micro-surgery, with the arm of the laser attached to the microscope. Off the microscope was a tube, down which I could focus the lens of the video camera I had taken along and which had been lent to me by a sympathetic TV & Video retailer. Through it, I could see into the child's throat and watch and record the laser at work as it cauterised the warts. I was told it had great advantages over conventional 'cutting' surgery – for the surgeon, greater precision down to the last millimetre and for the patient, no post-operative pain. The object of filming was to enable me to show people who contribute to the Fund, just what we do with their money.

'Weren't you squeamish, watching an operation?' is a question I was asked many times.

No, it was fascinating to watch, especially when it was helping a child.

Anyway, if you can pluck and dress a chicken with no problems, there was nothing to be squeamish about, for by comparison, the operation was a clean and tidy process.

The laser was the first of its type in a hospital in the North of England.

Another purchase by the Fund is 'Real time Ultrasound'. Many general hospitals have what is known as the B static mode ultrasound. Real time – a computer age expression meaning, 'as of now' is like the difference between still and ciné photography.

This also is now in use at the Christie and it is the first installation of 'real time' outside of London hospitals. At the time of writing, I haven't even seen it. Nor have we received the bill, which is likely to be in the region of £40–50,000. I know that Dr Eddleston, the Director of Diagnostic Radiology is delighted with it and that's good enough for me. An advantage is that, for some patients, real time ultrasound will yield the required information, thus leaving the sophisticated CT whole body scanner free to tackle more complicated cases.

I am increasingly reminded of that wartime slogan 'give us the tools and we'll finish the job'. If tools become available – and they undoubtedly will – which will help cancer sufferers, then I want them right there at Europe's largest cancer treatment centre – The Christie Hospital, which serves a North-West population of some five million people.

Some time in October I spent a typical day at the Christie – as usual, several appointments and also my medical.

My consultant examined me, giving my torso the usual prodding and pummelling.

'No change,' was his verdict.

'Are you going to start weaning me off the drugs, now that I'm on the countdown to the "five years cancer free" milestone?'

'No, that's not possible, Pat.'

'Oh? Why is that?'

'You've been on them too long. The drug has kept you cancer free, but a side effect is that your adrenalin glands are now inactive. You'll have to keep taking it for your source of energy.'

It had also caused a duodenal ulcer and I took another drug to keep that quiet! Now I understood why things seemed to require more effort than they used to do and why my consultant had made repeated attempts to get me to restrict my activities. And why my G.P. told me I'd no idea how to pace myself.

In the early days, the drug had given me an extra boost of energy in addition to my normal vitality. Now, it seemed, it was all I had left.

At first, the news deflated me. Then I told myself not to be a fool and to count my blessings.

I was still here, wasn't I? Still alive, still with my family, including the latest adorable addition, our little grandson David. I had so very much for which to be thankful. O.K. – so I would be taking drugs for the rest of my life. Was that so different from a diabetic who had to keep going on daily doses of insulin? And in any case, in view of that poor prognosis of six months, wasn't everything else a bonus?

Now I know the reason, I do try to conserve my strength. I do not – or try not to – take on more engagements than I can reasonably fulfil. If I know that I'm in for a late night attending a function or fund raising event, then I try to spend an hour 'horizontal' in the middle of the day. I may not sleep, but at least I am resting.

It is one of the reasons I had an Ansaphone installed. Another reason for having it is so that I do not miss people who may wish to help the Fund, or who ring to ask for help. For in the past three years I have had an ever increasing number of people – either cancer patients or their relatives – who want to talk to me, because they know they will be talking to a woman who understands the trauma that is cancer.

On the last day of September I visited Telephone House, Preston. It was not my first visit, for sometime previously, I had been entertained by the supervisors and staff when they had presented me with a substantial cheque, being the proceeds of a sponsored walk in aid of the Fund and in memory of a popular colleague who had died of cancer. On this occasion I was to receive a special telephone. On the following day the postal service and the telephone service were to go their separate ways. To mark the occasion of the in-

88

auguration of British Telecom, a limited edition of one hundred commemorative telephones had been made and I had been chosen as the recipient for this area. It was an honour indeed, for I daresay that eventually these commemorative 'phones will become collector's items. With it came a thousand free units for the Fund and I was invited to make a telephone call to anywhere in the world, using my new 'phone. Three-thirty in the afternoon in Preston and seven-thirty in the morning in Vancouver, so I had a five minutes chat with our friends Noel and Kay Beaumont.

My stainless steel telephone is press button and it incorporates the latest technology. I can plug it in at several points in the house, or if I am out, disconnect it and plug in the Ansaphone. It has since proved invaluable and is yet another example of the thoughtfulness and kindness I have received. During the course of the Appeal I have put some unlikely queries to the girls on Preston's telephone exchange. They have always been most helpful. If they could possibly find me the information I required, they have done so – and with the utmost patience and courtesy.

'Don't you find this sort of thing a drain on you?' I have been asked.

The answer is no, I don't, for if I am able to help someone else cope with it, then *my* day has not been wasted.

So let's take a look at some of the questions and I stress that the answers are purely my personal opinions as a patient. I am not a doctor.

First, should a patient be told that he or she has cancer?

Here, one cannot generalise. There are those who would die of a heart attack, or just give up at the very thought of having cancer. Others prefer to know the truth, whatever that truth may be, so that they know exactly what they have to face up to. It needs someone who knows the patient very well indeed, be it their doctor or a relative, to take the decision. And very often, having told them, they find they are confirming what the patient already suspected. My preference is for the truth, because it brought my family and me closer together, with no need for subterfuge or whispered conversations.

Secondly, the fear of death.

One could say every human being is dying from the day of birth. Each day that we live will never be lived again. It becomes a memory. By the same token, we cannot live tomorrow today.

Whether we are 100% fit or whether we are ill, tomorrow is a part of the future. Therefore, all any of us have is today. As for dying, we all do it. It is as natural an act as being born.

If we have a Christian Faith, we believe that we pass from this life into life everlasting. Then there are those who think that death is the end, with just nothing to follow. Why fear life everlasting? Why fear nothing? Therefore, why fear death?

Men and women are not just physical beings. We are also emotional, mental and spiritual beings. I believe that unless you are fighting cancer on all these fronts, you are not fighting it with the *whole person*.

Let me tell you a story which happens to be true. Two men, both cancer patients, were each given six months' expectation of life. The first man came home from hospital, went to see the local undertaker, made arrangements for his funeral and died a fortnight later. The second man, told to go home and put his affairs in order, looked at his seven children and thought 'What on earth will this lot do if I disappear from the scene?' Twenty years later, three of those children are now divorced and that man is *still* trying to put his affairs in order. What is more, he's crippled with arthritis! The reader is capable of drawing his or her own conclusions about that.

Then there is the fear of pain.

The old image of a cancer patient writhing in agony is out of date – or should be. Modern palliative treatment has reached such a degree of sophistication that even the terminal patient can be kept pain-free and mentally alert until a few hours before death.

Some cancer patients say that the treatment recommended for them is worse than the complaint. It may well be so. I remember feeling decidedly 'grotty' with no appetite at all and a weight loss of some three stones. But isn't it worth putting up with that – temporarily – in order that the cancer which might eventually kill you, should be either eliminated or controlled? And the old adage 'while there is life there is hope' is very true. Medical science and technology are advancing all the time. Great strides have and are being made in chemotherapy (drug treatment). When I was first a patient of the Christie in 1976 the five years cancer-free rate was under 50%.

Today, six years later, it is over 50% and that does not include those who might have reached that milestone had they not, in the interim, died of an accident or of a complaint other than cancer.

In trying to help cancer patients, I must have sent out – free – hundreds of copies of *One Day At a Time* and most recipients tell me they found it of comfort. Unfortunately, it is now out of print, except for the few copies I have retained for this purpose.

When you hit rock bottom there is only one direction in which you can travel – and that is UP! As the old song puts it, you have to 'pick yourself up, dust yourself down and start all over again.' It takes some doing, but it CAN be done, if you are prepared to fight with your whole being, every inch of the way.

Another Christmas came and went and at the turn of the year the total raised for my Fund topped the two and a half million pounds mark. That means that we have a balance in hand to keep the CT scanner updated as necessary and to purchase other technology as it becomes available. Yet because some of these items 'in the pipeline' may cost as much as the CT scanner, there will always be a need for money. As 1981 drew to a close, the Berkshire Appeal had raised £875,000; Lanarkshire £750,000; N. Ireland £635,000 and Stoke-on-Trent £440,000. All of them expect to have their CT scanners installed during 1982.

Our scanner at the Christie has now benefited over 2,000 patients. Among that number are the mother of Sister Doreen Woolley and the brother of Nurse Vera Feehan. Both of these dedicated nurses had looked after me in my darkest hours. As Vera put it 'It really is uncanny, for when you walked out of this hospital in January 1977, neither of us expected to see you again.'

I told her that she doesn't get rid of me that easily.

But in those early days the 'five-year cancer-free' milestone seems light years away. You think that if ever you reach it, you'll go out and paint the town all the colours of the rainbow. When it does happen, it's not like that at all. There is a feeling of quiet thankfulness coupled with the urge to reply to letters of congratulation with the words 'don't shout too loud – something may go wrong!' Yet I know that the publicity is necessary if I am to be of encouragement to other cancer patients and I know that recent TV, radio and newspaper coverage has been encouraging, for many people have written to tell me so. There have been so many kindly letters from well wishers in many parts of Britain – and an equal number of requests for help.

And yet, I am vulnerable. I say to Pauline as she sits typing, 'I hope all the people who have been praying for me and wishing me well don't suddenly stop.'

'I don't think they will, Pat.'

'That spiritual hovercraft has meant so much to me.'

They have been five action-packed years and at times I have felt as though I were in some kind of emotional tumble-drier and the support of so very many people has sustained me so very much. I know that my work has to continue. Being utterly selfish, I would like to return to full-time journalism. Yet I know I cannot. There are 350 patients in the Christie today and more will follow them, for the hospital sees 9000 new patients each year. I identify with them all. I understand their hopes, their fears, their anxieties and if I can work to help provide things which might help them, then this is the path I must follow.

A letter arrived at the Christie last month from a lady in Australia:

'Dear Sirs,

I have just lived, laughed and cried my way through *One Day At a Time*. Could someone please find the time to add a postscript to this story and let me know the current outcome of this lady's treatment and her work?'

The danger is, of course, that these pages will be compared with my previous book, which would be wrong, for it is the continuation of that story. I cannot be given a short time to live (heaven forbid) to start my Appeal all over again just for the sake of impact. But for those who like a happy ending, maybe it is encouraging to know that I am still very much alive.

To Miss Blackmore of New South Wales and to so very many people, I say, 'Thank you for your donation. Bless you all for your help. I couldn't have done any of it without your kindness, your good will and your support'.

9

AND NOW, FEBRUARY 1982 and that special holiday.

Years ago, when the Bishop of Lancaster and I were working for The Missions To Seamen – he was chairman and I was secretary of the Preston dock club committee – he said to me one day:

'Pat, my dear, I'll have to leave you to it for a couple of weeks. I'm taking a party of pilgrims to the Holy Land.'

With good humour tinged with envy, I had asked him if he needed anyone to carry his suitcase and had said that I had always wanted to visit Israel.

'Maybe I will get there someday.'

'You should, my dear. It's a profound experience and one you would appreciate.'

My beloved Bishop Tony was so right.

For here I sit on a greensward, savouring the peace of this lovely place. To the left is the Mount of Beatitudes and just a mile to the south is the city of Tiberias. In front of me the spring sunshine reflects on the tranquil waters of the Sea of Galilee. All is serenity and I reflect on the events of the past six years, beginning with a night in the Christie, during my first period of radiotherapy treatment. Unable to sleep, I had got up and gone in search of the ward kitchen and a cup of tea. With my usual aptitude for getting lost I had found myself in the kitchen of the children's ward where a friendly nurse and I had chatted over our tea. As I was about to leave, she asked if I would like to see the children. Tiptoeing past the cots and little beds I was filled with a cold fury that little children such as these should be stricken with cancer. Any self pity I might have been feeling went out of the window and along with the anger was a sense of helplessness. Oh, if only one could *do something* – but WHAT?

That night is indelibly printed in my memory and I suppose it is where the Appeal Fund began. Although it took several months and the added impetus of that six months prognosis to motivate me with a 'now or never' sense of urgency.

And so I had started to fight back, using whatever talent and experience I could call upon. I had asked, almost demanded, the help of other media men and women and that help had been gladly given.

They had helped to publicise my Appeal and a generous hearted public had responded magnificently.

The six month deadline came and went – and I was still alive. Oh well, maybe the medical people were a bit out in their estimate. Too soon to hope. In any case, I was now too busy to count the days. I was trying to live by my newly adopted discipline – one day at a time – and on days when I was feeling below par, it was damnably difficult to stick to it. Gradually, as my sick body began to regain some of its former strength, it began to be easier.

So busy, the time flew by. A year had passed. And then another and another. Crowded, eventful years . . . Could I now begin to hope? Why was I still alive? I was always an optimist, but was there more to it than just optimism?

I think that there was.

My mind goes back to April 1977 and to the little chapel of my beloved friend, Bishop Hoskyns-Abrahall, my 'Bishop Tony'. In this simple holy place I had brought all my trials to God, aware that they were as nothing compared to the suffering and the agonising death to which His Son had been subjected for the redemption of mankind. I had asked

Him to turn the experience of cancer to advantage for future cancer patients, so that my life and death should not be in vain.

Here are my troubles, Lord. Take them — and me — and use them as You will.

In that little chapel, Geoffrey and I had knelt before Bishop Tony, who had given me the Sacrament of the Anointing of the Sick. *Thou anointest my head with oil and my cup runneth over*. It was a most profound experience, almost impossible to describe. It was as though a kindly father, who loved me infinitely more than any earthly father could possibly love me, had affectionately ruffled my hair and said: 'I'm here. Don't be afraid. Leave the worrying to me, for there is work for you to do.'

All I know is that at that moment, the worry *was* lifted from me. My life and death were now in His hands and instead of fear there was trust and a new sense of purpose.

Later, Bishop Tony was to say: 'You don't always see miracles happen, but you know when they happen.'

Outwardly, I was still the same ordinary woman with a somewhat zany sense of humour and more than her quota of faults.

But as well as my new found peace and serenity there was now a singleness of purpose which made me drive myself remorselessly in pursuit of my objective, *knowing full well that I would be given the strength I needed*. I worked a sixteen hour day, week in, week out, dealing with mail, keeping appointments and travelling some sixty thousand miles in the process.

Through it all my husband Geoff supported me in every possible way he could think of. So did my family and friends. I owe so much to my mother and father, to my dear Pauline and my good friend Marie. Many is the time we have laughed together and sometimes cried together.

Then four years had passed since my consultant had called me into his office and had broken the grim news to me. Four years . . . was I going to make that five-year mile-

96

stone? May be now, I could really begin to hope . . . Optimistically, Geoff and I booked this special holiday and in company with forty-five other people it has been a pilgrimage. For us, a pilgrimage of thanksgiving.

What a good thing it is that we cannot see into the future, know what destiny has in store for us. Way back in May 1976 and that night when I had looked at those sleeping children, if anyone had told me of the events of the next six years, I would probably have died of fright, not cancer.

Here in beautiful fertile Galilee, did Jesus of Nazareth sit on this very hillside and, *knowing* His destiny, also know fear? I feel sure that He did and it is why he understands our fears and why He is ready to help us bear our burdens when we ask Him.

On the fifth anniversary of that day I walked out of the Christie with that fateful verdict, the first priority for Geoff and me was to visit Bishop Tony. We spent a quiet half hour with him in his study and with that special grace he has, he put into words all that I felt in my heart. Not only was I still alive, still with my beloved husband; I too, had witnessed a miracle.

A collective miracle of kindness and goodwill by countless men women, and children. It was truly riches beyond the dreams of avarice and a priceless jewel in a strife torn world. It was also the most humbling experience I could think of, for when human beings subjugate 'self' and work together for the common good, all things are possible. The Appeal had more than proved it.

And here, in this lovely place, where a certain Man told humanity to 'love one another' I am convinced that this is the ultimate Truth, for Love *is* the most powerful force on earth.

Years ago, Rome had impressed me because of its history and antiquity. For me, the essence of Israel is its timelessness, together with the thought that what a fleeting moment is a human lifespan.

Last week we were in Jerusalem. The Holy City, the hub

97

of Faith for three religions – Jews, Moslems and Christians. In its turbulent history, Jerusalem has been razed to the ground seventeen times but has always been rebuilt. It survives.

The massive walls of the old city are built of locally quarried pure white limestone which has mellowed to a magnolia colour with age. In the evening sunlight, they take on an apricot hue, which is no doubt where the writer of the hymn 'Jerusalem the Golden' found his inspiration.

Inside the old city, the scenes are much as they were thousands of years ago. Narrow streets through the souk, thronged with people, donkeys heavily laden and wares to be sold tumbling out onto the pavements . . . the smell of fruit and spices. The gradients are endless and steep, making it taxing for those who are fit. For me, with abdominal muscles 'cinderised' with radiotherapy, it was at times gruelling. Yet I was determined not to miss any of it. When we came to the site of Calvary within the Church of the Holy Sepulchre, the only way I could get up the final flight of spiral steps was on all fours. It was only later that it occurred to me that it was an appropriate way to approach the site of the Cross.

It was here that I offered to God the work of the last five years. Here that I gave thanks for my family and for my larger 'family' the men and women who are the local committees of my Fund. How I love them all. I gave thanks for their friendship and for the staunch support which they have unstintingly given to me. It was also a moment of rededication. I asked for the strength to continue the work on behalf of cancer patients; for patience and understanding to those who, facing cancer for the first time, ask for my encouragement.

During ten years as a Sunday School superintendent, I tried to use the skills of a journalist to make biblical events 'come alive' for the children. I talked about the people of places such as Bethlehem, Bethany, Jericho, the arid Samarian and Judean wildernesses, the Dead Sea. Now, at nearly fifty-four years of age, I have seen them all.

It was in the shepherds' fields outside Bethlehem that we sang my carol 'Brightest Star of Highest Heaven', the words of which are included in *'One Day At a Time'*. I could never have imagined when I wrote those words that one day they would be sung in the place where it all happened. Nor could I have imagined that I would be asked to read the Epistle in St George's Cathedral, Jerusalem, or that it would be that well loved passage from the 13th chapter of St Paul's first letter to his friends in Corinth ending with the words: 'and there abideth three things, faith, hope and love and the greatest of these is Love.' These are memories that will stay with me as long as I live.

Here in Northern Israel we have visited the source of the River Jordan at Baniyas and I am bringing home a container of this pure spring water for the Christening of a very special baby.

My dear friend Marie lost her only brother last September. Patrick died of a sudden heart attack at the age of forty-four. His wife was expecting their third child.

On 24th January, Carol gave birth to a beautiful baby girl and when she is christened Bernadette Louise, it will be with Jordan water. In Nazareth I purchased a child's olive-wood rosary, for the family are of the Roman Catholic Church.

As I let the beauty of the scene before me seep into my soul, I think and ponder on the events which took place here almost two thousand years ago and of the Man whose teachings, sayings and miracles were recorded by the four gospellers. Two scenes in particular have special relevance. The time when the storm blew up on these now calm waters. Ominous waves had rocked the boat and the fearful disciples had wakened Jesus. When he calmed the wind and the waters, they had marvelled but he had rebuked them, saying: 'Why are you so fearful? How is it you have so little faith?'

Faith implies implicit trust, even when we do not under-

99

stand or cannot find an acceptable reason for what is happening to us. Faith implies that the Almighty knows far better than we know ourselves, what is best for us. As Jesus was to say later in the Garden of Gethsemane: 'Not my will, Father, but Thy will be done.'

It was here also in this lovely land that he said: 'Why worry about tomorrow when today has sufficient cares of its own.'

How true that is. From my own experience I know that it is fruitless to worry about problems — hypothetical or real — which we might have to cope with tomorrow. It is only on this day — here and now — that we can do anything constructive.

For the past is but memory. What is to come is that unknown quantity, the future. Tomorrow is and always will be, another day.

So be it.